THE ATHLETE'S BODY

Published by
J. P. Tarcher, Inc., Los Angeles
Distributed by
Houghton Mifflin Company, Boston

THE ATHLETE'S BODY

HOW IT WORKS
HOW TO IMPROVE IT
HOW TO FEED IT
HOW TO REPAIR AND
PROTECT IT

KEN SPRAGUE
WITH JOE JARES

ILLUSTRATED BY EVERETT PECK AND
DÆRICK GRÖSS

Library of Congress Cataloging in Publication Data

Sprague, Ken.
  The athlete's body.

  Includes index.
  1. Sports—Physiological aspects.   2. Athletes—Health and hygiene.
3. Physical fitness.   4. Sports medicine. I. Jares, Joe, 1937-   . II. Title.
RC1235.S668   613.7'1   80-54542
ISBN 0-87477-151-X   AACR2

Requests for such permissions should be addressed to:
J. P. Tarcher, Inc.
9110 Sunset Blvd.
Los Angeles, CA 90069
Library of Congress Catalog Card No.: 80-54542
Design by Jane Moorman and Cynthia Eyring

Manufactured in the United States of America

AL 10 9 8 7 6 5 4
First Edition

To Homer Sprague, Frank Furtado, and Bruce Bennett, in recognition of their years of dedication and inspiration and their contribution to making better athletes.

Acknowledgments

A sincere acknowledgment to Kirsten Grimstad and Peggy Kimball for their exceptional editorial assistance, which substantially added to the depth and coherence of this book. Under the most demanding conditions, they remained charming and contributing throughout.

Thanks to Dr. Robert Girandola and Pete Grymkowski for their assistance in ensuring the clinical integrity of the manuscript.

A big thanks to Dærick Gröss for the years of perseverance in developing illustrations essential to effectively augment the text.

Most importantly, a special acknowledgment to Donna Sprague, without whose hundreds of hours of research this book would not have been possible. And without whose loving support this book would have a greatly diminished personal value.

Contents

Introduction

In *Othello*, William Shakespeare had one of his characters say, "Our bodies are our gardens," and these gardens can be left "sterile with idleness or manured with industry." That was the Bard's poetic way of saying, "If we work at it, our bodies will be firm instead of flabby or scrawny."

More and more Americans are manuring their bodies with industry these days. Record numbers of runners are entering races of from six kilometers to twenty-six-miles-plus. (Aerial photographs of the start of the 1980 New York Marathon made it appear that the fourteen thousand competitors were a huge swarm of insects.) Pre-Little Leaguers who can hardly lift a bat are hitting balls off batting tees in the daytime, and their fathers are going crazy over slow-pitch softball at night.

And while participant sports boom, spectators keep flocking to arenas and stadiums and hiking the ratings of televised events. There used to be sixteen major-league baseball teams; now there are twenty-six. Pro basketball has grown from six to twenty-three teams. Sports have moved into Monday-night TV and even have a cable network of their own, ESPN. The NBC broadcast of the 1981 Super Bowl was watched by ninety-five million people.

There are many reasons for the growth of interest. A popular president, John Fitzgerald Kennedy, gave a high priority to physical fitness in the early sixties. At least two sports, tennis and jogging, became chic activities, surviving the ultimate fate of fads because they had more to offer than most and won thousands—perhaps millions—of permanent converts. Educational campaigns explaining the health benefits of exercise have put the message across.

One of the most exciting advances is age-group sports. Track and field and swimming have age-group meets and records, and tennis and golf even have senior professional tours for men who in most cases are no longer competitive on the regular tours. There are men and women in amateur tennis who are *anxious* for birthdays to arrive so they can move, say, into the age 60-64 singles and doubles and start over as "young" stars again.

I can't overlook another major factor in the American sports boom. It used to be that a large percentage of women seldom or never participated in sports once they were finished with high school gym classes. Now they are out of the house to play soccer, softball, basketball, and field hockey, run track, etc., in greater numbers than ever before. These numbers will increase, too, because high schools and colleges have been forced by the courts to provide equal athletic opportunities for girls and women. It is becoming more and more acceptable for females to compete, use their muscles, and sweat.

The effects of the boom are all around us. Karate studios and athletic-shoe stores in the shopping centers, "sports medicine" an accepted specialty, "exercise physiology" an accepted research field, kids flocking to myriad sports camps run by such highly qualified people as ex-UCLA basketball coach John Wooden.

Just as important as the health aspect are the fun and excitement sports bring to us. This book is intended to fill the need for a layperson's reference source on all aspects of sports physiology in a way that conveys the fun and excitement of participation. The nougats of knowledge are candy-coated with humor and anecdotes from the lives of the stars—sort of like a blending of Henry Gray's *Anatomy of the Human Body, The Guinness Book of Records,* and the sports page, with cartoons thrown in for good measure.

The book is divided into four main sections: How It Works, How to Improve It, How to Feed It, and How to Repair and Protect It. To make things easy to find and easy to digest, the four sections are in turn broken up into short, simple essays covering everything from adrenaline to caffeine, from peripheral vision to blood doping.

The book is naturally full of bone and sinew, but it is no rival to Gray's *Anatomy,* nor is it meant to be. In these pages the bone and sinew are usually attached to a breathing, sweating, and sometimes hurting person—more specifically, to an *athlete.* When ligaments are up for discussion, pitcher Tommy John's ligaments illustrate the point. When it's sore knees, basketball player Julius Erving's aching pair provides the example.

My hope is that after digesting the information presented here, and putting in some hard work, athletes will find that their bodies look better, feel better, and *are* better. May their gardens bloom.

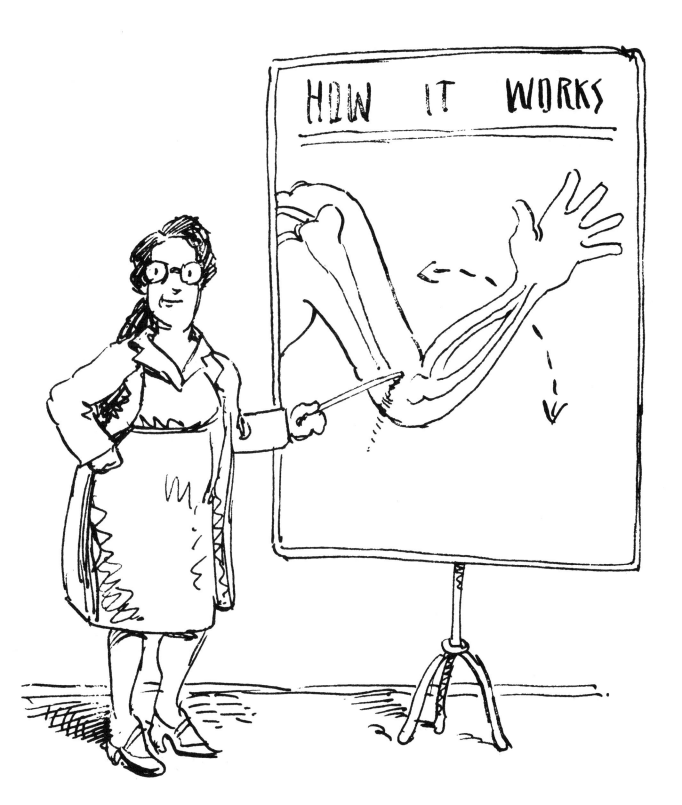

Introduction:
All Systems Are Go

*T*he human body is a complicated contraption. It takes in and processes fuel. It gathers, sorts, and acts on information. It recreates itself (with the cooperation of a body of the opposite sex). It sleeps, dreams, breathes, feels pain, thinks up jokes, fends off germs, cools itself, cries, and, most important in this section, moves. Moves not just in mundane ways—walking the dog, sitting down, stirring the soup—but in ways that give pleasure to both mover and observer. In ways that give benefits, too.

Dancing is an example. And athletics. When we're admiring the grace and skill of a soccer player controlling the ball with his feet, we can't see the myriad systems at work inside him. Messages flash along his nerves, glands secrete hormones, blood delivers oxygen to his cells. He is a wondrous, flesh-covered bag of guts and gases, muscles and bones.

The body is worth only a few pennies if broken down into its chemical components, but it's priceless if it has the gift of thought, of movement, of life. Then it can get off the launching pad with all its interconnected systems working efficiently.

Let's examine those systems that are important to athletes.

The Motion System

Skeletal Muscles: The Primary Movers and Shakers

Tom Seaver winds up and throws a sweeping curveball past the batter. Strike three! Nothing to it for a big, strong guy like that, right? Wrong. Seaver uses approximately fifty different muscles to toss that curve. These muscles interact to pull on the bones of the upper arm and forearm, creating the twisting forward thrust that gives spin to the ball. And that's not counting his leg kick and long stride toward the plate.

Complicated athletic motions require the synchronization of many muscles acting on the same or several coordinated pairs of bones. No wonder it takes years of practice to become a major-league athlete.

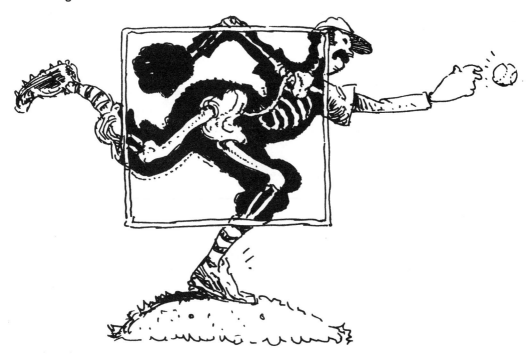

There are several types of muscles, but the skeletal muscles are the primary movers and shakers in sport. Each skeletal muscle is attached to two bones. Each pair of bones, pulled by its common muscle, produces the basic athletic motions: running, reaching, jumping, bending, and so on. The stronger and faster the muscles move their pairs of bones, the better the athlete performs.

Skeletal muscles are connected to bones by tendons—usually one tendon at each end of the muscle. The tendon acts as a bridge between the muscle and the bone, and the muscle's force travels across this bridge as it pulls on the bone, creating motion.

Inside Seaver's body, muscles, bones, and tendons collaborate like dancers in a well-rehearsed ballet to create motion that is smooth, effective, and pleasing. Of course, the opposing batter rarely appreciates this artistry.

Muscles' Teamwork

Biceps   Triceps

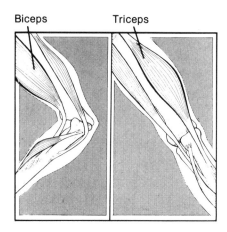

Fig. 1. *Bending or straightening the elbow requires the coordinated interplay of bicep and tricep.*

A pair of muscles works much like John McEnroe and Peter Fleming in a doubles tennis match: when one partner is on offense, the other is setting up the defense. When one muscle contracts (draws together) to move a bone, the other relaxes, allowing the bone to move.

The biceps and triceps of the upper arm are an example of the pairing of muscles. The biceps is the large muscle at the front of the upper arm that bunches into a hard lump when someone "makes a muscle." (Lou Ferrigno, TV's Incredible Hulk, has a twenty-three-inch biceps, and twenty inches is not unusual in bodybuilding.)

The triceps—the muscle at the rear of the upper arm—works in tandem with the biceps, as shown in Figure 1. When the biceps contracts to bend the elbow, the triceps relaxes and allows the bend. When the triceps contracts to straighten the arm, the biceps in turn relaxes. If the two don't cooperate, there is a standoff. The elbow stays locked in position until one of the muscles yields from fatigue or injury.

The cooperation of the biceps and triceps is typical of what takes place throughout the body. When entire groups of muscles get involved, the interaction simply becomes more complex. For example, the forward thrust of a Chicago Bears linebacker requires the simultaneous contraction and relaxation of hundreds of muscles in the legs, back, shoulders, and arms. For the brain, muscles, and nerves, it's like the difference between choreographing a Fred Astaire tap-dance solo and an entire musical show.

Were You Born with the Right Muscles?

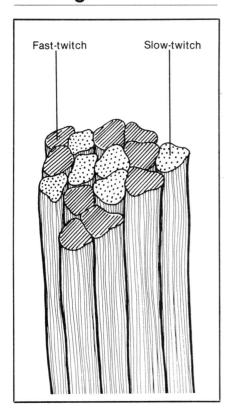

Fast-twitch   Slow-twitch

Fig. 2. *Fast-twitch muscle fibers help speed the sprinter to the finish line, while slow-twitch fibers provide energy reserves for the marathoner.*

Muscles can be different in composition as well as size, and that composition difference can determine the kinds of sports for which you're best suited. It's all a matter of twitches.

Hair color, eye color, and skin pigmentation are physical characteristics we inherit from our parents, as are such components of athletic ability as height and bone length. These features are obvious, but other, less obvious inherited traits have an even greater influence on athletic performance. The makeup of muscle tissue is an example. Muscle tissue is composed of groups of similarly functioning cells banded together in fibers.

Exercise physiologists, who specialize in the body's response to exercise, have shown that skeletal-muscle tissue is composed of two types of fibers: fast-twitch and slow-twitch (see Fig. 2).

Slow-twitch fibers can store more glycogen—a form of stored carbohydrate that is the muscle's energy source. Thus slow-twitch fibers enhance performance in endurance events such as distance runs, since the more energy stored in the muscle, the more energy the runner has available to endure the run.

Fast-twitch fibers, on the other hand (or foot or leg), affect both speed and strength, so they are important to sprinters and weight throwers. In fact, the *quickest movements* of any athlete at the 1956 Olympic Games were made by 350-pound Paul Anderson, the heavyweight weightlifting champion. This was verified by videotape analysis.

Everyone has both fast-twitch and slow-twitch fibers, but in different proportions. An athlete might have 80 percent slow-twitch fibers and 20 percent fast-twitch, which would help him in marathons and hurt him in sprints.

The proportion is determined at birth, and no kind or amount of training will change it. If you're born with 80 percent slow-twitch fibers, you'll go to the grave with that percentage, and you'll never be a good sprinter.

An athlete can reach his *personal* muscular potential through training, but, like the color of his eyes, his potential in strength or endurance events is determined by his parents. Some athletes are naturally gifted; some aren't.

There's only one way to find out your proportion of fast-twitch and slow-twitch fibers: through a microscopic analysis of a small amount of surgically removed muscle tissue, usually from a large muscle group such as the calf. Keep in mind that positive results might be a head start toward success, but having the right tissue doesn't replace the need for hard work.

Marathon Man

There is little doubt that when slow-twitch fibers were passed out, Jay Helgerson was near the head of the line. Helgerson is a marathoner, one of those all-lungs-and-legs masochists who compete in races 26 miles, 385 yards long. Since he is in his mid-twenties and in perfect health (at least physically), his choice of sport isn't too unusual these days. What *is* unusual is that early in 1980 he completed an unprecedented feat: running in and finishing fifty-two marathons in fifty-two consecutive weeks.

He started January 28, 1979, in Saratoga, California, and finished January 19, 1980, in Houston. He finished all but seven of the marathons in under three hours except for the two *ultra*marathons in his itinerary—a fifty-miler ending in Sacramento and a thirty-one-miler in Davis, California.

Well, let's be absolutely honest. On Saturday, March 24, he ran a marathon in Bakersfield, California, in 3:23. Disgusted, he drove north to Davis and on Sunday did 2:57.50 in the Run for Life Marathon.

"I just threw Bakersfield out," he said. "I figured, 'This is what's fun about this. Since it hasn't been done before, I can make my own rules up as I go along'."

Helgerson wasn't always such a well-oiled and durable machine. He didn't compete in any varsity sport in high school in Wichita, Kansas, where he grew up, and in fact he couldn't even make the ninth-grade basketball team. His first run of any distance was three miles in combat boots—while going through Marine basic training at Parris Island, South Carolina.

He ran his first marathon in June of 1975 while still in the Marines. He had been jogging about five miles a day but had

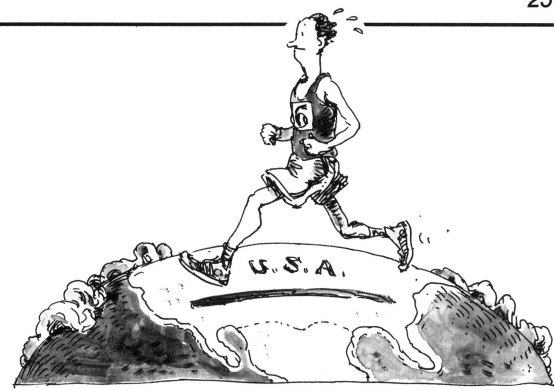

never gone more than ten. At twenty-two miles of that first ordeal, his calves were hurting so much that he sat down on the curb and, shielded from the oncoming runners by a parked car, cried.

Before starting his year-long odyssey he had completed forty marathons, twenty-five in one year. In his "fifty-two" year he took on just about every kind of terrain and weather condition possible in North America. In Grandma's Marathon, from Two Harbors to Duluth, Minnesota, he had a lovely view of Lake Superior to his left the whole way. In Pinole, California, he tackled Pig Farm Hill ("You're going straight up, practically, with your knees just missing your chin"). At the Cowtown Marathon, Fort Worth, Texas, it was five degrees below zero with the wind-chill factor, and runners were slipping and sliding on the ice. In the blistering heat of Omaha he ran the last six or seven muggy miles with his perforated shirt over his head to block out the sun.

"There definitely were weekends when it was tough," Helgerson said. "I kind of got down. But the thing is I didn't get pushed into it; nobody had a knife at my back. It's something I wanted to do. It was my Olympics, my Superbowl."

What Makes a Muscle Grow?

Famous bodybuilder Arnold Schwarzenegger has a fifty-eight-inch chest and a twenty-two-inch biceps, and, as you might guess, he didn't simply order his spectacular muscles from a mail-order house or have them grafted on. It took planning and hard work.

Muscles grow through a combination of exercise and a nutritious diet. The exercise stimulates the growth that nutrients in food make possible. If the muscles are properly exercised, they will grow on any balanced diet.

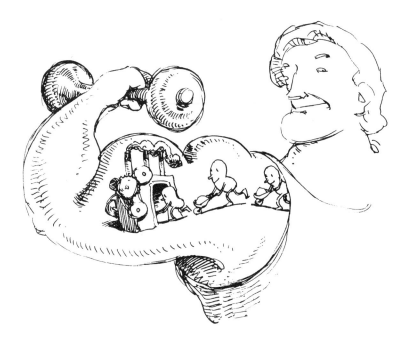

Of course, this regimen of exercising and eating is a simplification of the process through which muscles grow—a process that is still not entirely clear to scientists. One theory is that when a muscle encounters resistance, the resulting contraction causes production of a chemical called creatine. In turn, creatine stimulates the formation of myosin, the protein directly responsible for muscular contraction. These two chemicals have a spiral effect on muscle growth: a contraction creates creatine, which causes formation of more myosin and a correspondingly stronger contraction, which will produce still more creatine, and so on. The result: bigger and stronger muscles.

The best way to exercise for muscle size is to place continually greater demands on the muscles during workouts. This concept is usually called progressive resistance training (discussed later in the section on "How to Improve It"). As the muscles become capable of handling a given demand, the demands are increased. Weightlifters use this method when they systematically lift heavier and heavier barbells. These increased demands require stronger muscle contractions, which, in turn, promote growth. It's the practical application of the contraction-creatine-myosin cycle.

The Case of the Shrinking Muscle

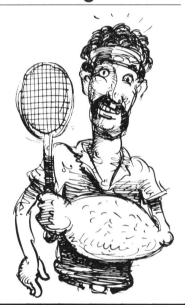

Australian tennis player Rod Laver has a huge left forearm, developed to Popeye proportions not by spinach but by months and years of forehands, backhands, serves, and volleys. Yet if Laver should give up tennis and turn to chess, the size of his forearm would soon start decreasing.

Like a polio victim or a patient coming off a two-week bout with the flu, an athlete who doesn't use his muscles allows them to shrink and weaken. In fact, the level of conditioning is affected by as little as a two-*day* layoff, and two months of lollygagging will go a long way toward nullifying the effect of years of training.

The athlete's body looks—and usually is—a lot healthier than the average person's, but the two bodies are subject to the same unforgiving laws. Bodies marshal forces where most needed. And when Rod Laver is not practicing or competing, his strong forearm isn't necessary. The body phases out the extra muscle tissue in an extremely complex chemical process. Therefore, many athletes train during the off-season, when a little effort will protect most of their muscle gains and allow them to begin the competitive season in strong condition.

Can the Female Athlete Grow Big Muscles?

Stand at poolside at a national-championship meet and look at any top female swimmer—Tracy Caulkins, Cynthia Woodhead, superb butterflyer Mary T. Meagher—and you will see a pair of broad shoulders. This supports bodybuilder Arnold Schwarzenegger's statement about women's muscles: "They grow larger from being trained and fed, just as men's do."

However, Caulkins, Woodhead, and Meagher could follow Mr. Universe around the weight room duplicating every arm curl and squat, yet never come close to developing his bulk. The reason is their body chemistry, specifically their short supply of testosterone.

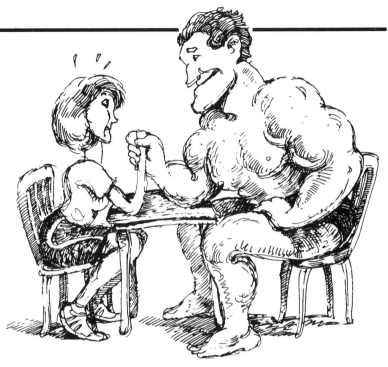

Testosterone is not an Italian dessert but an essential hormone that promotes muscle growth. It occurs in significant quantities only in male bodies. Females don't have enough of it to grow bulging, man-sized biceps.

Male athletes have long used synthetic testosterone derivatives to increase their hormone balance and accelerate muscle growth, but its role is not as simple as it might at first appear. Recently a number of women have experimented with testosterone injections, with mixed results. At least some women saw no improvement (evidently it is not this hormone alone that accounts for the complex muscle-growth cycle). Yet at recent female bodybuilding contests the muscular development of the competitors—a few of whom were known to have aided their natural processes by hormone hanky-panky—has been truly amazing. (Playing games with hormones can be dangerous for either sex. See "How to Improve It: The Steroid Struggle.")

In addition to more testosterone, men have the mechanical advantage of proportionately longer muscles stretched over longer bones. Many female athletes have doubled their strength through several months of weight training. In fact, women usually gain strength through weight training faster than men. This may be due to the fact that women have demanded less of their muscles before discovering the delights of barbells, thus allowing greater potential for improvement.

Mr. America or a Vogue Model— Who Has More Muscles?

Posing under a spotlight and slathered with oil, Mr. America seems to have steel slabs and cables bulging and rippling under his skin. But he really has no more muscles than a *Vogue* model who looks as if the next suggestion of a breeze would sweep her away. Everybody, male or female, is born with approximately six hundred muscles, from the large ones of the back, arms, and legs to the *stapedius*, one-twentieth of an inch long, which controls a tiny bone in the middle ear.

Muscles can be made stronger and bigger, but you can't grow new ones. They can be made to grow by increasing the demands placed on them, as bodybuilders and football linemen do by hefting weights. In fact, Mr. America of 1978, Tony Pearson, added more than seventy pounds of muscular bulk to his body.

We may all have the same number of muscles, but heredity, training, and, yes, sex combine to determine how big and powerful they will become.

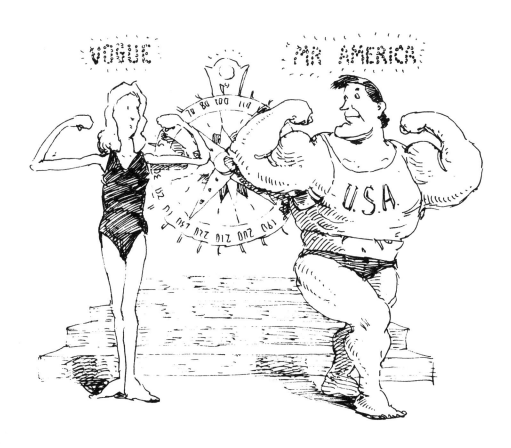

Inactivity: Swivel Hips to Hippo Hips

Lots of people believe that those big athletic muscles developed through a grueling training regimen will turn into hog lard when the exercising stops. Absolutely not. Muscle is muscle and fat is fat; neither will change into the other.

When the athlete quits training, muscles shrink and a layer of fat forms over them. Why? Simply because active Mr. Swivel Hips, the All-America running back, becomes inactive Mr. Hippo Hips, eating more than he needs for energy (Fig. 3).

When the athlete is in training, he develops eating habits to match the energy demands of that training. This could mean an extra three thousand calories a day. If he doesn't cut down when training, he'll daily be putting away three thousand calories more than he burns. That's about six pounds a week!

The extra six pounds are stored on the body as fat—not in place of muscle, but over muscle in such places as the skin, stomach, and rump. The muscle is still there, but you can't see it through the suet.

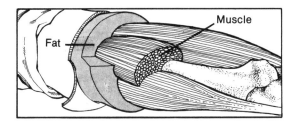

Fig. 3. *Eating in excess of your energy requirements causes a layer of fat to form on top of (not in place of) muscle.*

It's no secret that fat can get out of control. The fattest man who ever lived, according to the *Guinness Book of World Records*, was Robert Earl Hughes of Illinois. He got up to 1,069 pounds in 1958 and died of uremia soon after.

On the other side of the coin is Charles White, USC's Heisman Trophy-winning tailback in 1979, who was tested by the school's physical education department and found to have only 1.94 percent fat in his 183.7-pound body. The measuring technique, which involves immersing the subject in water, has a 2-percent margin of error high and low.

Dr. Robert Girandola, who often conducts such tests in a big wooden tub in the PE building basement at USC, estimates that the average running back has 9 to 10 percent fat, the average college-age male about 15 percent, and the average offensive-line behemoth about 20 percent.

The Body's Connectors

Fig. 4. *Tendons and ligaments hold the body together, tendons connecting muscle to bone, ligaments connecting bone to bone.*

On July 17, 1974, Los Angeles Dodgers Pitcher Tommy John ruptured a ligament in his left elbow. Two months later Dr. Frank Jobe, an expert on sports injuries, performed an interesting operation—robbing John to pay John, so to speak. He removed a seven-inch strip of tendon from the pitcher's right forearm and, according to the *Los Angeles Times*, twisted it "into his left elbow in the hope that the body would accept it as a ligament."

Well, the body certainly did. John returned to the mound for the Dodgers and the New York Yankees. On the sixth anniversary of the surgery, late in the 1980 season, his new pitching arm had a record of ninety wins, forty-one losses.

Ligaments and tendons often come into the sports spotlight, usually because of injuries like Tommy John's. Not all stories have such a happy ending.

Ligaments and tendons are the body's connectors. Tendons hold muscles to bones, and ligaments hold bones together, as illustrated in Figure 4.

Ligaments are made of strong, pliable tissue, much like very tight, strong elastic bands. They need pliability to allow joints to bend, and they need strength to withstand the tremendous force placed on joints during movement (for example, force placed on the knee during a jarring football tackle or the repetitive force absorbed by the knees and ankles during a jog).

Next time you're preparing chicken, examine the whitish material that holds the bones of the wings together. This will give you an idea of what human ligaments are like.

Ligaments respond to the stress of exercise by growing thicker and stronger. Stretching exercises help to make them more pliable, allowing the joint a greater range of motion.

Tendons, which are found at either end of a muscle, serve as the intermediary between the muscle's contraction and the bone's motion. The number of tendons attaching the muscle to a bone determines the name of the muscle. For example, a biceps (*bi* meaning two) has two tendon attachments at the bone, a triceps has three, a quadriceps four.

Tendons respond to the stress of exercise in the same way as ligaments and muscles: they grow thicker and stronger. And the tendon-bone attachment becomes correspondingly stronger as well, helping prevent the tendon from being torn away from the bone by a strong muscle contraction.

Bones Thicken from Athletic Stress

Athletes put more stress on their bones and muscles than most people, and bones respond to this increased stress exactly as muscles do: by getting bigger.

If you would love to add a few inches in height—say, to increase your chances for basketball stardom by growing from a midget into a six-foot-ten-inch center—don't get your hopes up. Bones grow *thicker*, not longer, from stress. Those bones that receive the most stress add the most thickness, particularly the hips (pelvis) and thighbones (femurs). Imagine the stress on hips and thighs when a basketball player comes down with a rebound or a halfback tries to break a linebacker's tackle.

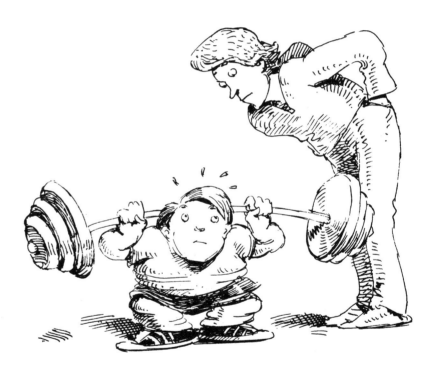

Bone response to stress is the reason many doctors warn against heavy, strenuous weight training for pre-teenagers. They believe too much pressure placed on a still-growing skeletal structure could stunt growth or do other harm. Although no definite evidence has been found to support this theory, it should be considered when dealing with a young athlete.

Black Athletes: Color Them Fast

You would have to be blind not to notice that black athletes are prominent and often dominant in most of the major sports. *Sepia* magazine reported that twenty-four of the medals won by American track-and-field athletes in the 1976 Olympics were won by blacks. And all the U.S. gold medals in boxing were won by blacks. Of course, there are sociological reasons for this—there is a saying, "White boys grow up wanting to be President, and black boys grow up wanting to be Willie Mays." Because of racial discrimination, sports is one of the few avenues to greatness open to black youngsters.

There are physiological reasons as well. Blacks, on the average, have longer arms and legs, shorter trunks, narrower pelvises, denser (therefore heavier) bones, more muscle in the upper arms and legs, less muscle in the calves, less muscle overall, more tendon, and heels that don't stick out as much.

Most of these attributes are athletic pluses and explain in part why the majority of America's best sprinters, basketball

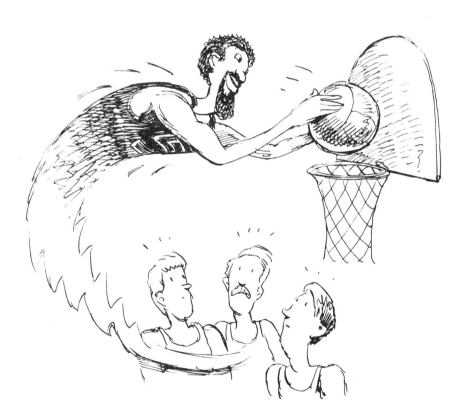

players, and long jumpers are black. The heavier bones might explain why so few swimmers of quality come out of black neighborhoods; blacks tend to be "sinkers." (Sociological factors creep in here too, though. Few black neighborhoods have swimming pools and swimming clubs.)

All human beings (except albinos) have dark pigmentation, or *melanin*, in their skin. Blacks obviously have more of it than whites. Various physical-education experts around the country, including Dr. Malachi Andrews of California State University, Hayward, and Dr. Lee Edelstein of the University of California, Davis, are looking into melanin as a possible reason for blacks' superiority in sports.

"Until recently, melanin had been thought to be a fairly inert [powerless, without motion] pigment," said Dr. Edelstein, "and that it wasn't terribly important except for its ability to protect the skin from harmful effects of the sun such as skin cancer or rapid aging. But now people have gotten interested in melanin because the pigment can absorb a great deal of energy and yet not produce a tremendous amount of heat when it absorbs all of this energy [from the sun]. Therefore, it's conceivable that it could be transforming this harmful energy into useful energy."

Much more study must be done. But perhaps melanin is the reason, for instance, that in a 1978 track meet, black sprinters took forty-eight of forty-nine places in three sprinting events: the 100-, 200-, and 400-meter dashes.

The Cooling System

The Body's Thermostat

Every fall there are instances of high-school and college football players dying during or after practice in hot weather because their athletic pads and clothing have caused too much internal temperature buildup. Even *without* clothes and pads, intense exercise can elevate the body's temperature beyond 105 degrees F.

Our bodies operate best at the normal temperature of about 98.6 degrees F. Everyone who has had a fever knows how bad a rise in our body temperature makes us feel: weak and clammy, unable to perform such routine chores as vacuuming or typing a report. The higher the fever, the worse the effects. If the body's temperature rises more than ten degrees above normal, the protein structures of the brain and organs start to break down and slowly cook.

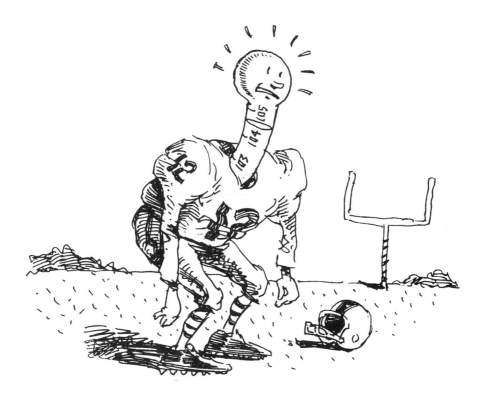

Going the other way on the thermometer, a drop in body temperature below 96 degrees F. causes the cellular enzymes, particularly in the brain, to become less active. Ten degrees below normal and the heart stops.

If your body had a motto, it might be, "Save the core at all costs"—either from a meltdown while you're exercising in warm weather or from letting your internal organs turn into Popsicles in cold weather. Changes don't have to be so dramatic to affect the athlete, however. Minor temperature changes—less than two degrees—can have major effect.

Our nerve signals depend upon the diffusion of molecules through the membranes of the nerve wall. And this diffusion rate is affected by temperature. A change of several degrees in body temperature rates can cause erratic nerve impulses. Simply put, the brain responds to the temperature change by signaling the muscles to contract too early or too late. The athlete's timing is destroyed. Instead of hitting a home run off a favorite pitch, a feverish Reggie Jackson's nerves miscalculate and he strikes out.

Athletes Are Hot-Blooded

Julius Erving romping up and down the basketball court for the Philadelphia 76ers, Nadia Comaneci spinning around the uneven parallel bars, you or the paunchy guy next door pushing a lawnmower uphill—when people exercise vigorously, their muscles put out energy at the same rate as a three-hundred-watt light bulb. But muscles are not efficient, so most of this energy doesn't go into motion. In fact, about 70 percent goes into *heat* energy, and, if there's no heat dissipation, you get hotter. Exercise at the rate of three hundred watts could raise the temperature of a 150-pound body about six degrees per hour.

Let's take a science-fact (rather than science-fiction) voyage inside Erving's body. Since some of this heat is trapped within, his interior and his muscles get hotter than the surface of his body. If there was no way of quickly removing much of this excess heat from his innards, his temperature would steadily go up until he was forced to the bench or even to the hospital. He cannot allow heat to accumulate. But when operating smoothly, his body does get rid of this excess heat energy.

Heat will not move easily from the interior to the body surface because muscles, organs, and tissue are poor conductors of heat. (Remember how long it takes to cook the middle of a roast.) So nature has come up with a solution: using a liquid—Erving's blood—to carry heat energy away.

Blood is mostly water, which is a glutton for heat and soaks it up at a much greater rate than other materials do. *Thirty times* as much heat can be absorbed by a pound of water as by, say, a pound of copper with the same resultant rise in temperature. And since Erving's blood is mostly water, it has a great capacity to absorb heat. ("Hot-blooded" should be used to describe athletes, not Don Juans or people with bad tempers.)

The hot blood flows to the surface of Erving's body, where it fans out into the many miles of tiny blood vessels called capillaries. At the same time, his brain signals his skin to sweat more. Why?

Only a thin layer of flesh separates the sweat forming on the surface of the body from the miles of heat-filled capillaries just below. (See Fig. 5.) This allows Erving's blood to transfer its heat easily through the skin to his sweat. His cooled blood then flows back to the interior to pick up another load.

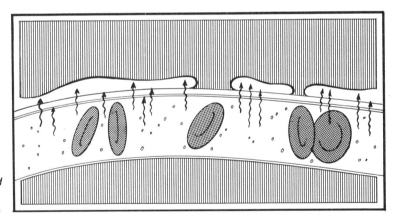

Fig. 5. *Capillaries carry the heat produced by exercise from the muscle tissue to the skin surface, where it evaporates as sweat.*

The heat doesn't stay on the sweaty surface of the body. If it did, the surface would be unable to cool the next load of hot blood. At this point another property of water comes to the rescue: it can evaporate. And evaporation carries away the heated sweat.

Your cooling system works just like Julius Erving's, continuing night and day. You usually don't notice the process—after all, there's no air conditioner humming. But when you exert yourself, evaporation can't keep up with the internal heat output, and the accumulation of sweat is the telltale sign.

Dressing to Keep Cool

When you're sitting in the fiftieth row of a football stadium on a hot September day, it might appear that the players on the grass below are wearing solid cloth jerseys. But if you were down among them you'd see that the jerseys have so many holes they look almost like nets. The holes are escape routes for heat.

To make the most of your cooling apparatus, it is best to wear loose-fitting clothes or no clothes at all. With too much clothing, there is no air circulation at your skin. The cloud of water vapor stays near the skin and effectively stops any more evaporation, and sweat without evaporation is useless as a cooling method.

Consider a similar situation with a heated pan of water. Imagine gently heating the water well below its boiling point. Some of the heat from the burner will raise the temperature of the water, and some of the heat will change a portion of the liquid to a gas of water vapor. The invisible vapor will carry away the heat which formed it. The water will eventually reach some steady temperature and stay there while it slowly evaporates. But what happens if you cover the pan?

With an airtight cover on the container, the evaporated water will have no place to go, thus halting further evaporation since there is no unlimited atmosphere into which the vapor can flow. Almost all the heat will then go into raising the

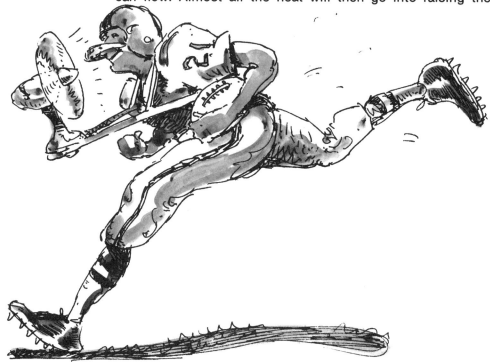

temperature in the covered pan, and the pan will get hotter and hotter, just as the body gets hotter and hotter under tight clothing.

So bare skin is better, and a cool or even warm breeze across the skin is better yet. The breeze blows away the hot vapor cloud as soon as it appears above the skin, making it easy for more evaporation to take place. The whole process is speeded up. This is similar to blowing across the surface of a hot cup of tea. The hot gas just above the tea's surface is blown away, speeding up evaporation and cooling the tea near the surface a little.

How about swimmers? Well, of course, like anybody else, they sweat when they exercise vigorously. And if the pool water is warm, they'll sweat more. But much of the heat is washed away instead of departing via evaporation.

"It Ain't the Heat, It's the . . ."

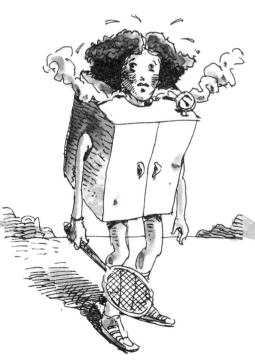

It's no coincidence that Houston and New Orleans have enclosed, air-conditioned stadiums (the Astrodome and the Superdome, respectively), because those cities are among the most humid in America. There are summer days in New Orleans when you can get almost as wet strolling through the French Quarter as you would swimming in Lake Ponchartrain.

Playing football or just carrying out garbage cans is a miserable chore in hot, humid weather. Heat alone isn't bad for the athlete. The body can stand dry heat of 200 degrees F. for several hours without a significant loss in efficiency. It's humidity that prevents the exercise-generated heat from leaving the body fast enough. Sweat rolls down your body and soils your clothing rather than evaporating.

In humid climates, evaporation is prevented because the atmosphere is already saturated with water. For example, 50-percent humidity means that the air contains 50 percent of the water it can possibly hold. On such a steamy day, your body's cooling system can operate at only 50-percent efficiency, working just as hard as usual but with only half the results. At 100-percent humidity, the surrounding air can't accept any more water (sweat) and your body's cooling system is operating with near-zero results.

Endurance activities are affected most by humid conditions. It's not unusual for a distance runner to collapse from the combined effects of heat and humidity. The internal heat generated by the continuous running rises and rises until a heat stroke hits. The same thing frequently happens during summer football drills. The football player trains in hot, humid weather with the added heat insulator of heavy clothing, which keeps the heat in, not out.

Athletes compensate for tropical, sweaty days by shortening practices and wearing fewer clothes to allow for better ventilation and evaporation. The rest of us compensate by loosening our ties and postponing the garbage duties.

The Disadvantage of Not Being a Camel

As we've already seen, exercise produces body heat, which sweating (called perspiration outside the locker room) removes from the body. So sweating is an important part of the body's marvelous cooling system. But a problem arises when the body sweats too much: dehydration, or loss of water.

Anytime the body has less than its maximum water level, it's considered dehydrated. Of course, the degree of dehydration matters. A drop of water lost isn't noticeable. Losing even a quart of water won't hurt much. But loss of a gallon might cause serious problems for the athlete. And during strenuous exercise on a hot day, water loss can be as great as a gallon per hour!

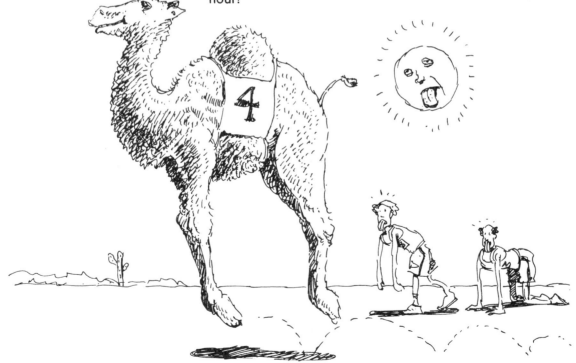

Just a 2-percent weight loss from dehydration (for a 150-pound athlete, that's three pounds, or one-and-one-half quarts) affects the efficiency of the nervous system by raising body temperature above 100 degrees F.

An 8-percent weight loss produces an internal temperature of 105 degrees F., a higher pulse rate, and symptoms of dizziness and nausea.

A 12-percent weight loss can result in permanent loss of motion by halting the operation of the brain and heart.

Dehydration affects all body systems, particularly the circulatory. The blood thickens from the water loss, and more strain is placed on the heart to pump this beet-soup mixture through the arteries. Although this is the time of greatest need, less food and oxygen are carried to the energy-starved cells to replace the energy expended through the exercise. The bottom line is a plunge in cardiovascular efficiency.

Experienced athletes drink continuously during hard exercise to counterbalance dehydration. However, the body can absorb only about a quart of water each hour. That's why athletes remain thirsty for a long time after exercise; the body is trying to repay the water deficit.

Dr. David L. Costill, director of the Human Performance Lab at Ball State University in Indiana, recommends that athletes doing hot, hard work should drink fluids *before* feeling thirsty and should avoid sugared drinks, which are slow to be absorbed from the stomach.

It's unfortunate that people don't have the same resistance to dehydration as the camel, which can lose as much as 25 percent of its total body weight through a decrease in its water supply without *any* fluid loss in the blood itself. This is possible because—as recent studies by a Duke University physiologist and an Israeli zoologist have shown—camels don't store water in their humps, but conserve it in their nasal passages. These passages, tiny and winding, are moistened by glandular secretions, which form an absorbent crust as the animals lose water. "This crust soaks up moisture coming from the lungs," reported *Time*'s science section. "During inhalation, the stored moisture is carried back into the lungs." Thus, since camels store water in this auxiliary tissue and dissipate it from there rather than from the bloodstream, their blood supply is not diminished by water loss. People, on the other hand, lose water from all available sources, including the bloodstream.

In a marathon, bet on the camel.

Making Weight at the Last Minute

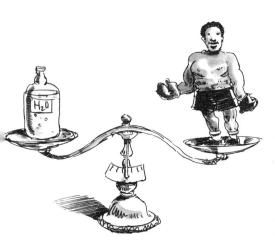

The scale shows that he's eight pounds overweight. The weigh-in is tomorrow. It's too late to diet because that much weight can't be lost that quickly through dieting. The only way to make weight is to dehydrate. But he can't afford the bad effects on nerve impulses, strength, or endurance caused by a substandard water balance. Can he lose the water weight for the weigh-in and regain it before the competition? Here's how one Mr. World solved that problem.

Mr. W took a common prescription diuretic (which increases urination) during the twenty-four hours before the weigh-in. He lost eleven pounds of water. To replace the minerals lost through dehydration, he took mineral tablets, particularly potassium, throughout the same twenty-four-hour period. After the weigh-in, he drank water to regain the lost fluid and restore his body's balance.

Mr. W's system could work for any athlete who has to make weight at the last minute. Is it unfair to opponents who get their poundage down without the help of gimmicks? You bet! But, although doctors generally regard this practice as both foolish and dangerous, many athletes *do* dehydrate for competition weigh-ins. And this can create a considerable weight advantage.

For example, weigh-ins at boxing and wrestling tournaments usually occur six to eight hours before the bouts begin. During larger tournaments, the weigh-in might be earlier than that. Hence the middleweight can dehydrate eleven pounds for the weigh-in and regain the lost fluid during the day. He'll have an eleven-pound weight advantage when he steps into the ring.

Disadvantages of the dehydration method, however, include cooling-system problems (e.g., overheating) and electrolyte and body-salt imbalances. These conditions can lead to premature fatigue, muscle cramps, and lightheadedness—all of which, though not life-threatening, can severely impair athletic performance.

Generations of athletes have made weight by spending hour after hour in a steam room or running around the auditorium. Light-heavyweight boxing champion Victor Galindez, a bull of an Argentine, lost his title to Mike Rossman in 1978 and put part of the blame on the two days he had to spend in a sweatbox to make the weight.

Unfair though it may be, many athletes are accomplishing the same weight "adjustment" with just a few swallows.

Competing in Eskimo Weather

When exercising in a gym, arena, or enclosed stadium, there is no danger of becoming too cool. But some sporting events are held outdoors in sled-race weather conditions—cold, wind, and snow. Late in the pro football season it's common for the Minnesota Vikings to play home games on what resembles arctic tundra. Their bodies must deal with these gelid conditions by taking steps to keep warm when they are losing too much heat.

But how do their bodies lose heat in the first place? Even when they're surrounded by cold air, if adequately clothed they don't lose much heat by evaporation. They lose most of it by warming the cold air they breathe and by passing heat through their pants, pads, and jerseys to the outside air. These heat losses eventually will reduce their internal heat to a dangerously low level if left unchecked.

In response to too much heat loss, bodies take both defensive and offensive measures. The first line of defense is to reduce the size of the surface blood vessels, blocking the escape of heat through the skin. When bodies shut down surface blood vessels, hands become stiff and less sensitive. Viking receivers have to warm their hands on the sidelines to counteract this effect, or they'll have difficulty hanging onto passes.

The body's major offensive measure is to burn more food to generate more internal heat. Reducing the size of the surface vessels while increasing the rate of food-burning is analogous to closing the windows of a house and turning on the furnace. One without the other is useless.

Remember that motto of the body, "Save the core at all costs." And if it has to remove blood from the surface while burning more food, it will do so. Normally, the measures described here are enough to supply the body's heat needs.

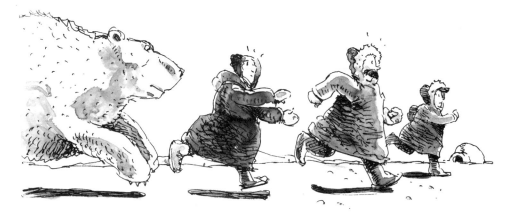

But if heat loss continues and the core continues to cool—let's say you've fallen off your sled and are lost in a Yukon blizzard—the body goes into its last-ditch defense against incapacity: it shivers.

Shivering is a series of rapid muscle contractions, or "quivering." Most of the energy produced by a contracting muscle is heat energy, which will heat the core. So quivering muscles are really internal heaters. But shivering is only a short-term emergency heating system. If rescue doesn't come or if shelter isn't quickly found, shivering soon exhausts the last of your energy and you cool off. Permanently.

The Right Way to Take a Shower

Various cities around the country have Polar Bear Clubs, with members who go swimming in Lake Michigan or some other icy body of water in the dead of winter and at least *pretend* to enjoy it. An athlete who has just had a strenuous workout should leave such stunts to polar bears.

Take a look at yourself after a long, hard training session. Your heart is still pounding as the sweat forms on your skin—sure signs that your internal temperature remains high from the recent activity. Now ease under a stream of water slightly cooler than your body's temperature. Your touch is your thermometer. The water temperature nearly matches your body's, so there is no shock. As you feel your body cool, gradually cool the water until your body's temperature is normal.

Why not just jump under the cold water? Because the sudden blast of coldness on the skin confuses the body's cooling system. Many heart attacks have been brought on by the Finnish custom of going from a sauna (a steamy, hot bath) into the snow and back into the sauna. You can imagine the shock to the heart and circulatory system caused by that routine.

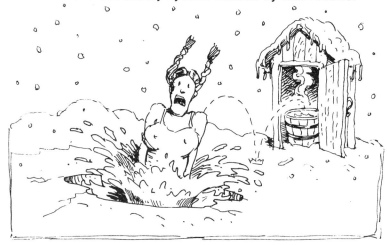

The Energy System

Energy: From Sun to Cell

Operating a power saw, heating the house, or blocking an opposing lineman requires energy. Where does this energy come from?

Almost all the energy we use on earth originated as sunlight, which shines on plants and is captured by their fibers in the form of radiant energy. The plants are in turn absorbed (eaten) by animals. Buried animal and vegetable matter then decays under hundreds of thousands of years of extreme compression, which eventually turns it into oil and coal. Thus the coal we burn to generate electricity and the high-priced oil we use to operate the family car are really stored sunlight!

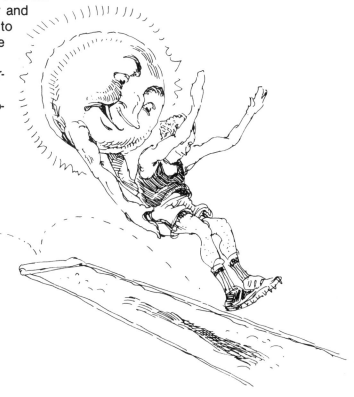

Similarly, we can generate hydroelectric power only because sunlight evaporates water to be dropped later as rain, causing the rivers to flow. The flowing rivers, most notably the Colorado, turn the hydroelectric generators.

The source of all our bodies' energy is sunlight too. But we cannot directly convert sunbeams into human vigor; if we could, sun-worshipping nudists would be walking power-houses. As we've seen, however, plants *can* take energy directly from the sun, so for our energy supply we eat plants or we eat other animals that eat plants.

After we eat to supply our energy needs, the nutrients must still be routed to the muscles, bones, and organs via the bloodstream.

The bloodstream doesn't just aimlessly flow along like a meandering creek. The right food is delivered to the right destination, just as if there were a busy traffic controller stationed in the brain or heart. For example, if an athlete's muscles need quick energy during a discus throw, it will be drawn directly from the energy stored within the muscles themselves. But if the need is less immediate, as in a short, steady jog, energy is supplied to the muscles by the delivery of oxygen through the bloodstream. If the demand is not at all urgent, such as a need to gradually restore energy to fatigued muscles, the energy comes from the liver, where it has been stored for later use. Finally, an additional energy source is the fat cells, to which the bloodstream has routed excess food energy for long-term storage. (The fat deposits are essentially a reserve food supply, tapped only when too little food is consumed to meet the body's energy demands.)

In short, the bloodstream is a remarkable remote-control energy stream. It channels oxygen from the lungs and nutrients from the stomach to the cells, where they are combined to produce life-giving energy.

The Athlete's Unromantic Heart

I Left My Pump in San Francisco and *My Pump Belongs to Daddy* are songs that probably wouldn't even make a hydraulic engineer's hit parade. But the heart, celebrated by lyricists and storytellers as the body's headquarters for courage, generosity, sympathy, and love, is really an unromantic, hard-working pump made of muscle.

This workhorse of an organ weighs about half a pound, yet it recirculates your six quarts of blood more than two thousand times a day. Each day of your life it pumps more than twelve thousand quarts of blood—three thousand gallons, or enough to fill a tanker truck—through the more than sixty thousand miles of blood vessels in your body. The yearly volume circulated by the heart amounts to enough blood to fill three huge oil storage tanks or a supertanker.

The heart—already the strongest muscle in the body—can grow bigger and stronger just as other muscles can. All of them respond to progressive resistance training, in which demands are gradually increased.

After a runner achieves a five-minute mile, he attempts to run even faster to place increased demands on his strengthened heart muscle, and it tries to pump even more oxygen through stronger beats. The runner should remember that muscle growth takes time. He can't strengthen his heart with a few days' running any more than Woody Allen can grow big biceps or bench-press four hundred pounds after a week in the gym. To attain good results, the runner should put in at least fifteen minutes of aerobic exercise per day over a sustained period of time.

There are significant differences between the unconditioned heart and the athlete's heart.

A NORMAL HEART:

Is the size of a fist.

Pumps with the same force it takes to squeeze a tennis ball.

Pumps seventy-two times a minute.

Beats one hundred thousand times a day.

THE CONDITIONED, ATHLETIC HEART:

Is larger and stronger than the normal heart (see Fig. 6).

Beats fewer times a minute (thirty to thirty-five beats a minute is not an unusual resting rate, and tennis star Bjorn Borg's is only twenty-seven).

Beats fifty thousand times fewer each day than the normal heart; it's an energy conserver.

Supplies oxygen-filled blood to the body with half the effort of the normal heart.

Has enlarged arteries—two to three times larger in diameter than normal—to accommodate the increased blood flow.

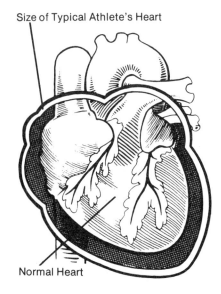

Size of Typical Athlete's Heart

Normal Heart

Fig. 6. *The enlarged, conditioned athlete's heart improves general functioning as well as athletic performance.*

Success in most sports events is dependent on the heart's capacity to pump oxygen-filled blood. Strengthening the heart enhances the performance of general activities as well as athletics, and it helps prevent heart attacks. Many doctors a generation ago thought a bigger, "athletic" heart was something bad—not much more welcome than a goiter or tumor. Now the medical profession overwhelmingly endorses the health benefits of a stronger, bigger pump.

Hemoglobin: We Deliver

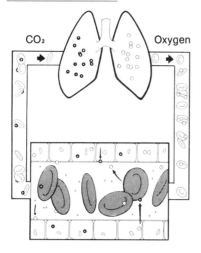

CO₂   Oxygen

Fig. 7. *Hemoglobin transports oxygen from the lungs to the cells for energy production and carries away the waste products in the form of carbon dioxide.*

Blood takes its color from the red corpuscles suspended in the blood fluid. These red corpuscles are the body's oxygen carriers. More precisely, oxygen is carried by a chemical compound within the corpuscles—hemoglobin. Oxygen passes through the walls of the blood vessels of the lungs and into the bloodstream, where it combines with the hemoglobin.

The bloodstream then carries the hemoglobin along until it reaches the cell wall. Here, the oxygen is freed from the hemoglobin and passes through the cell wall into the cell body, where it transforms food into energy.

No less important than its oxygen-carrying job is hemoglobin's other assignment for the cells. In every cell in the body, "burning" food and oxygen create a harmful byproduct, carbon dioxide, which must be eliminated. Like oxygen, carbon dioxide easily attaches to hemoglobin.

The process is then reversed. Carbon dioxide created through the oxygen burn goes back into the bloodstream, combines with the hemoglobin (which has released its oxygen), and is carried to the lungs. After it gets back into the lung tissue, it's exhaled into the surrounding atmosphere. Having dumped the carbon dioxide at the lungs, the hemoglobin is ready to pick up another load of oxygen. The cycle, depicted roughly in Figure 7, then repeats itself.

Blood Doping

At the 1972 Olympics in Munich, Finland's Lasse Viren won the five- and ten-thousand-meter runs, a very difficult double. He had many poor and mediocre performances after Munich, yet he came back at the 1976 Olympiad in Montreal and won the same two races again.

At that time there were widespread rumors—denied by Finnish officials and Viren himself, and unproven to this day—that his victories had been accomplished using an experimental technique known as blood doping, or injecting extra blood into the athlete's body prior to competition. (Other runners who attempted to benefit from this technique did not achieve notable success, however, and the practice has since been denounced on both practical and ethical grounds.)

Red blood cells carry oxygen from the lungs to the body's cells. And adequate oxygen delivery is the foundation of endurance activities—a category that certainly includes Viren's events. So does injecting the athlete with extra red blood cells help his performance? The evidence is inconclusive, but people still try it. Here's how.

Four to eight weeks before competition, a doctor withdraws a large amount (as much as a quart) of an athlete's blood. The doctor then separates the liquid (plasma) from the red cells. The red cells are refrigerated and stored.

By competition time, the athlete's body has replenished its natural blood supply. The doctor then injects the red blood cells that had previously been removed. The effect is that the athlete then has a higher concentration of red blood cells and, consequently, a greater oxygen-carrying ability. The appeal of this technique for the cheat is that no drug or illegal substance shows up in any post-event test.

There is little doubt that the increased concentration of red cells carries more oxygen. But there is a detrimental trade-off. Thickened by the increased concentration of red cells, the blood is harder to pump, causing greater strain on the cardiovascular system. More oxygen is delivered, but at a greater energy expenditure.

The potential for unfair competition using this method is great. Swedish physiologist Bjorn Ekblom carried out an early blood-doping experiment with seven students in 1971. "I am not interested in creating supermen," he said at the time. "I am frightened at the possibilities of its [blood doping's] use within sport."

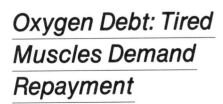

Oxygen Debt: Tired Muscles Demand Repayment

As you're reading this book, your muscles are being supplied with oxygen by your bloodstream. The oxygen burns with carbohydrates and fat (from digested foods) to give the muscles the energy it takes to sit erect and turn the pages.

The same principle applies to the athlete. As he or she covers mile after mile on the road, track, or playing field, the blood supplies oxygen to the muscles to be burned with carbohydrates to manufacture the energy necessary to place one foot in front of the other time after time. The waste products of

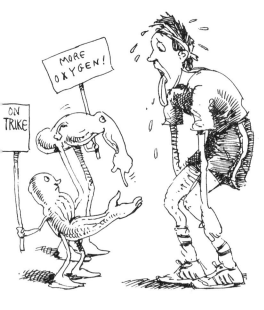

this oxygen-carbohydrate burn—water and carbon dioxide—are safely and quickly eliminated from the body. Everything is going smoothly.

But what happens in an emergency? Say the apartment catches fire, and you have to run down fifteen flights of stairs to escape the flames. Unless you're in great condition, your legs will be screaming in pain as you wait for the fire truck to arrive. Your situation is similar to that of the distance runner who must leave a comfortable pace, shift into overdrive, and sprint the last quarter-mile to the tape. The runner, too, is in pain from the unexpected muscular activity. Why?

The exertion required more oxygen for the muscles involved than the bloodstream could supply. Without that oxygen, the muscles had to create their own energy source. They used glycogen, an energy reserve that's stored within each muscle. Glycogen needs no oxygen to produce energy. But the breakdown of glycogen produces a harmful waste product—poison, in fact—lactic acid.

The muscle can only stand a little lactic acid. That's why tiredness sets in and you feel pain within the muscle. The accumulation of lactic acid must be stopped and indeed reversed. But removal of it requires oxygen. That's why you and the runner keep panting and gasping for air after your emergency run. The panting will continue until you have given the muscle enough oxygen, via the bloodstream, to break down and haul away the lactic acid. In other words, the panting continues until you have repaid the "oxygen debt" owed those tired, painful muscles.

Extra Blood for Working Muscles

When a battle breaks out at a corner of a fort, the commandant no doubt will send extra legionnaires racing to help at the trouble spot. Similarly, the body will send more blood to pitcher Ron Guidry's arm when he's on the mound facing opposing batters than when he's sipping a leisurely cup of water in the dugout.

Automobiles, light bulbs, and muscles use streams to deliver energy. Depending on the system, that energy is provided in the form of gasoline, electricity, or blood. It is each stream's responsibility to deliver as much energy as needed. The more "juice" required, the more gas, electricity, or blood delivered. Of these three systems, the bloodstream is the most complicated during times of heightened demand.

Let's take our pitcher, Guidry, as an example. The first step in increasing delivery of blood to his arm muscles is for the heartbeat to quicken, pumping more blood into his arteries. But to help his muscles, the blood must enter them, so the muscles' arteries and capillaries open wider.

About five teaspoons of blood per minute enter each pound of Guidry's resting muscle. But when a muscle works hard—as the muscles of the wrist, arm, and shoulder certainly do in pitching—as much as *seventy-five* teaspoons per pound enters through the widened arteries and capillaries. This extra blood means extra vim.

What causes the blood vessels to widen? Simply put, Guidry's working muscles release potassium, phosphate, and lactic acid. And, like a chain reaction, these chemicals cause the smooth muscles lining his vessels to relax, thus allowing them to open up.

At the same time, the vessels in his nonworking muscles and internal organs constrict (reduce in diameter). In fact, Guidry's liver and intestines lose as much as 80 percent of their normal blood flow while he's trying to put his opponent's clean-up hitter back on the bench with a strikeout. He needn't worry, though, because those organs at rest need only 10 to 20 percent of their normal energy supply.

This ability of the bloodstream to route more energy to areas of need while largely ignoring resting areas is yet another example of how the body works to keep balance.

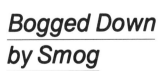

Bogged Down by Smog

Smog is the ugly, eye-smarting haze that hangs over Los Angeles and other metropolises. There are hot summer days when high-rise buildings just down the block are almost invisible. The smog is so pervasive that residents are startled when, after a windy night, they walk outside in the morning and can actually see the beautiful mountains that partially ring the city.

Many industrial, car-clogged cities have smog, but the phenomenon has reached its greatest infamy in L.A., which will be the site of the 1984 Olympics. September is the worst month for polluted air, so Games planners have wisely scheduled the track-and-field events in the downtown Coliseum for late July and early August. However, even during those months the air there is not known for its Rocky Mountain purity.

How does putrid air affect athletes? No conclusive evidence is available, but most authorities see smog as a menace to athletic competition.

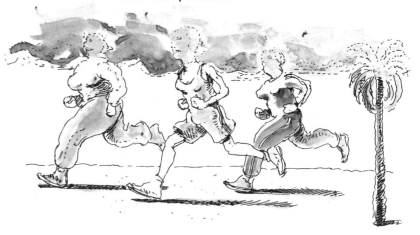

"Air pollution has disastrous effects on performance, particularly in endurance events, where the athlete relies on oxygen flow," says Dr. Walter Jekot, a sports medicine specialist.

"Certain combinations of heat and smog could create a disaster, and I'm talking about athletes keeling over in long-distance events," says Dr. Stanley Rokaw, an L.A. lung specialist. "Symptoms would include acute chest pain, breathing difficulty, and burning eyes.

"We need more research in this area, but we can't find anyone to fund it. We have a good idea how ozone and carbon monoxide affect athletes, but we have no data yet on how PAN (peroxypropionyl nitrate) affects athletic performance. PAN is a chemical agent peculiar to L.A. smog."

Carbon monoxide gushing from car exhaust pipes is a common threat, especially to those running on or near roads. Why is it dangerous? Dr. Jekot: "Red blood cells prefer to bond with carbon monoxide rather than oxygen. In fact, this preference is greater than two hundred to one. This causes the needed oxygen to be left behind in the lungs while the useless carbon monoxide is carried around by the red blood cells."

Ozone, also common in L.A. and elsewhere, is a big hindrance. As little as .5 part ozone per million in the air can cut down cardiovascular performance by as much as 10 percent.

It's not uncommon for L.A. to record ozone levels five times *higher* than that. So don't look for great marathon times in '84.

"Stay away from roadways and try to work out during times when pollution is less, " warns Dr. Jekot, "usually during early-morning and late-evening hours when fewer automobiles are on the road. Lighten your training effort on a very smoggy day or you risk injury to the cardiovascular system."

The Body Feeds on Itself

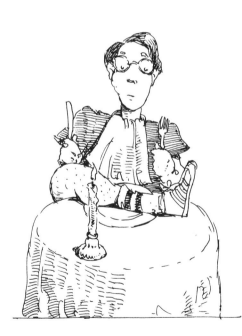

Runner Jay Helgerson, the fellow who finished fifty-two marathons in fifty-two weeks, can burn as many as twenty-five hundred calories during a race or workout. During the rest of the day he might burn another twenty-two hundred just grocery shopping, taking out the garbage, and doing other mundane chores. Let's say his total energy expense for a day is forty-seven hundred calories. He has eaten foods containing forty-two hundred. How can he burn five hundred more than he consumes? Energy has to come from somewhere, so his body feeds on itself. There's an internal cannibal in all of us.

When the body has used up the energy from recently eaten food, the next source tapped is stored fat and glycogen. Fat and glycogen are taken first because they are more easily converted into energy than protein. This daily consuming of the body's stored fat is the method of weight-loss diets.

A conditioned athlete is at or near ideal competing weight, so he or she doesn't want to follow the dieter's pattern. It is important for the athlete to monitor calorie intake to match the outgo. This is best done by frequent trips to the scale. It doesn't take many days of intense training and careless eating to burn away a half-dozen needed pounds. And the lost pounds may not be all fat.

It is not uncommon to find a finely tuned athlete with as little as 2 percent body fat. What happens if that 2 percent of fat is entirely consumed by the body because the athlete hasn't been eating enough? The body begins to feed on its own muscle tissue for energy. Then the problem is serious. The least that will happen is loss of muscle efficiency as the athlete heads toward the pathetic image of a person suffering from malnutrition.

Generally, doctors recommend that athlete and non-athlete alike keep a little body fat "hanging around" for emergencies (about 10 percent). The rationale is that it's safer to carry around a few excess consumable pounds than to take the chance of burning muscle that has taken months or years to build. However, many athletes roam the fields and courts healthily with less than 5 percent body fat.

Adrenaline: The Competitive Juice

When Chris Evert Lloyd gets ready to start a tennis match her body goes on alert, and crucial changes occur: her heart starts thumping quicker and harder, and her blood pressure rises. You might say her competitive juices are flowing. Those juices are blood and adrenaline.

What is adrenaline? It is a hormone that is released from Lloyd's adrenal glands (above her kidneys) and is greatly increased when play begins. It is not known what triggers the increased secretion of adrenaline in Lloyd and the rest of us, but it is probably related to psychological effects and the nerve reflexes in the cardiovascular system.

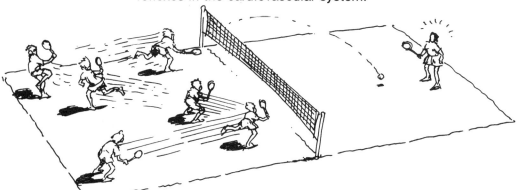

Studies do point out that almost at the split-second Lloyd hits her first serve, the concentration of adrenaline in her blood increases. And when she moves around the court to hit her accurate ground strokes, adrenaline causes her heart not only to beat faster but also to contract more forcefully, thus pumping more blood with each contraction—up to six times as much as at rest, approximately thirty quarts a minute! This increased blood flow is helped by the dilation of her coronary arteries, which is also caused by the adrenaline.

During a match, adrenaline also aids in energy production by speeding up the conversion of glycogen (an energy source in the form of a carbohydrate stored primarily in the muscles) to glucose (an energy source traveling through the bloodstream) and thereby raising Lloyd's blood-sugar level. This extra blood sugar is needed by her working muscles, and as soon as the blood reaches the widened capillaries of those muscles, the blood pressure will decrease and return to normal.

Adrenaline is also responsible for inhibiting intestinal movement during performance, allowing the athlete's blood to be diverted from the stomach and liver so that more blood will flow to working muscles.

As soon as Lloyd has won the match point and her body cools, adrenaline decreases to its pre-exercise blood level.

The Nervous System

The Body's Switchboard

Along with all the other wondrous goings-on inside your body—glands secreting, arteries dilating, cells receiving regular deliveries of food and oxygen—there are messages flashing back and forth with enough speed and accuracy to make Bell Telephone and IBM jealous. Accepting, delivering, analyzing, and responding to messages are jobs handled by your nervous system.

The basic component of this communications network is the "neuron," which is the technical name for the nerve cell. A neuron is like a single telephone line, with a transmitter at one end and a receiver at the other. (See Fig. 8.) The transmitter telegraphs vital as well as trivial messages along the line to the receiver.

Many telephone lines can be packed inside a single cable. And likewise, many neurons can work side by side inside a single sheath of tissue, each neuron carrying its own message.

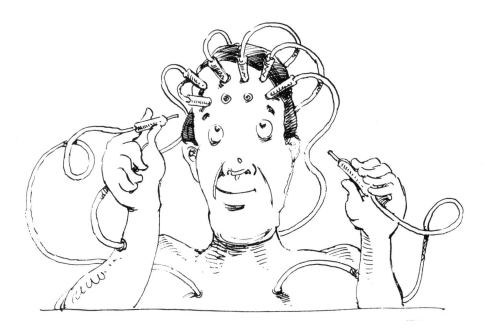

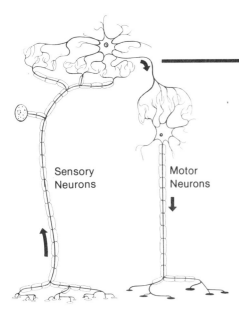

Fig. 8. *Sensory neurons transfer messages to the central nervous system, where they are analyzed and then responded to by motor neurons.*

Like the signals along a telephone line, messages zipping along the neurons are electrical. If you feel, see, or hear something, neuron sensors in your skin generate small electrical voltages—signals that are transmitted along the neuron pathways to your brain.

Some of the millions of neurons that compose the brain analyze the meaning of the electrical messages it receives. This analysis occurs when neurons in the brain exchange information among themselves. They form computer-like circuits allowing you to think. After the brain determines the right response to the incoming information, it sends a return message along other neuron pathways, calling for the reaction—a swimming stroke, a leap, a head fake, a kick.

Success in sports is tied to how well the neurons do their jobs: how fast they pick up messages, evaluate the information at the brain, and make appropriate responses. And the speed and precision with which small-voltage messages are generated, transmitted, and processed by neurons are affected by many factors, which we'll examine in the next few articles.

The Human Computer

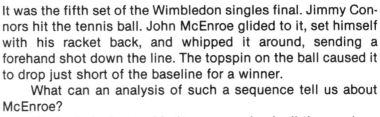

It was the fifth set of the Wimbledon singles final. Jimmy Connors hit the tennis ball. John McEnroe glided to it, set himself with his racket back, and whipped it around, sending a forehand shot down the line. The topspin on the ball caused it to drop just short of the baseline for a winner.

What can an analysis of such a sequence tell us about McEnroe?

His brain had stored in its memory bank all the previous shots he and Connors had made. It knew what to expect. Before McEnroe's return shot, it stored and interpreted information such as: where Connors had to go to retrieve the previous shot, what shots he could be expected to make from that position, weather conditions at Wimbledon's Centre Court, McEnroe's own position. All those calculations happened before Connors even struck the ball. In other words, McEnroe knew the sport well, and his brain programmed itself.

As the ball left Connors' racket, nerve impulses moved from McEnroe's eyes to his brain, telling him the position of the ball. As the ball moved, nerve impulses continued to report changes in the ball's position. And McEnroe's brain sorted this information. As more information was processed, it predicted the trajectory of the ball.

As his brain interpreted the information presented to it, it sent a sequence of orders to McEnroe's muscles, which in turn sent him gliding off on the intercept path, set him up for the stroke, and caused him to strike the ball.

To play the game that well, McEnroe practiced long hours to gain experience. A brain without experience needs much longer to predict and respond to the flight of the ball. Indeed, for beginners, most responses have to be thought out consciously. With experience, the motions become automatic because the brain has calculated the correct response before. So McEnroe does many things on the court automatically. He has spent the time needed to program his computer.

As James Gregg says in his book *The Sportsman's Eye,* "Incoming images are matched with what is on file. The better the file, the more accurate the interpretation will be."

Tissue Remembrance

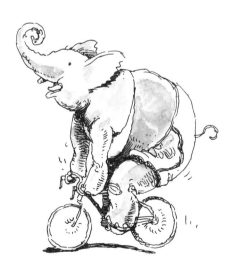

Watch a child learning to write. Getting the mind and fingers to work well together often takes several years of practice. The same holds true for developing athletic techniques. Years were needed for golfer Al Geiberger to perfect his fairway shots and for batting star George Brett to perfect his swing. But once developed, the skill can be neglected for months or years and then quickly reacquired, at least in part.

The reason is tissue remembrance. The tissue, whether muscle or nerve, has a memory bank that stores the previously obtained information. In, say, Geiberger's case, particular nerve patterns necessary to duplicate that fluid golf swing are retrieved from the billions of brain cells.

Nerve responses are quickly sharpened in the first training drills. In fact, the nervous system must wait for the muscular system to catch up with its re-education. That takes a little longer. But once that level of conditioning has been reached, the athlete is at top form once again.

Famous bodybuilder Arnold Schwarzenegger took many years to sculpt his body. For a movie part he had to lose approximately twenty pounds of his hard-earned muscle tissue, which he did. What is remarkable is that he regained all that muscle within six weeks of resuming hard training!

Professional football players combine both muscle and nerve remembrance. After the off-season layoff they come to training camp slow, weak, and rusty. But almost miraculously, within a few weeks, they play ball as pros are expected to play. They keep their jobs through tissue remembrance.

In the Blink of an Eye

A bumblebee near the face, sudden bright lights, or a fighter's punch causes a reflex blink. Can the reflex—a natural protective response—be controlled by the athlete? Yes.

Successful boxers learn to eliminate blinks during competition. If they didn't, that split-second blink, called "glove shyness" in the ring, would leave the boxer vulnerable to a surprise punch.

Eliminating the blink, or any reflex, is accomplished through practice. In the boxer's case, a conscious effort is made to keep the head forward and the eyes open amid flying punches. After a week or so, the repeated conscious effort becomes natural as the blinkless eyes stay fixed on the opponent.

Volleyball players also learn not to be gun-shy. A novice player might leap to block a spike and close his eyes at the moment the opponent hits the ball. A veteran such as UCLA All-America Karch Kiraly will jump at the net and—he hopes—unblinkingly watch the rival's spike bounce off his blocking hands.

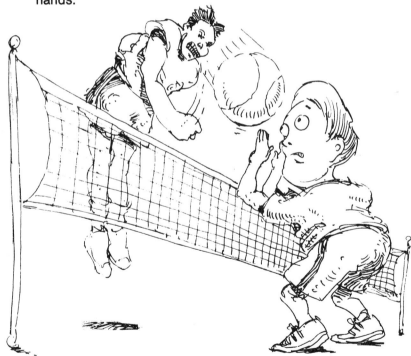

Keep Your Eyes on the Ball

Pass receivers are told again and again by coaches that they must "look" the football into their hands. When they forget this lesson and glance around for tacklers or turn toward the goal before the ball is safely caught and tucked away, they often drop perfectly thrown passes.

"Everyone has good hands," says Pat Tilley, a pass receiver for the St. Louis Cardinals, "but the important thing is eye-to-ball coordination. After the pattern is called and the ball is thrown, that's the job—to get out there and catch it.

"I like to spend time practicing one-handed catches. There's nothing better to sharpen the concentration. I don't practice them that way so I can make them in a game. I do it to force myself to keep my eyes on the ball."

This is true in other sports too. The shortstop is supposed to watch the baseball plop into his glove and only then look toward the place where he's going to throw it. A tennis player is admonished to look at the ball as it bounces off his racket strings. Tennis coaches are always yelling things like, "Read the label on the ball" or "Keep watching the spot where you hit the ball."

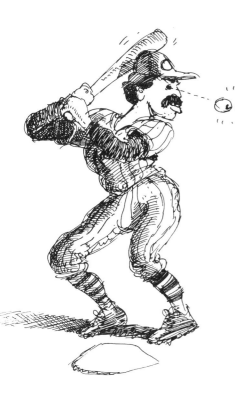

Similarly, a batter strives to see the baseball hit his bat and fly off. Considering that some pitchers can throw fastballs a hundred miles per hour or more, that's not easy. But the batter isn't weaponless. Nerve impulses can travel up to 265 miles per hour, so his eyes and brain can work quickly indeed. Hall of Famers Babe Ruth and Ted Williams had extraordinary vision, which helped them become extraordinary hitters. More recently, Kansas City A's third baseman George Brett has been using his sharp eyes and concentration to torment pitchers.

". . . Brett has a talent for watching the ball all the way to the bat," says pitcher Jerry Koosman. "That takes intense concentration. Some hitters pull [their eyes] off the ball a foot or two before it strikes the bat, and that's the difference between a line drive and a foul ball."

Interestingly, it has been found that everyone has a *dominant* eye. Most right-handed people have a dominant right eye and most lefties have a dominant left eye, but, according to the Council on Sports Vision, about 20 percent of the populace has crossed dominance. That can be a big advantage in baseball.

The council tested 250 major-league baseball players from six teams and determined that about half had crossed dominance. The *Los Angeles Times* reported: "The council found players with crossed dominance have an advantage in picking up the flight of the baseball, since they can sight it from the proper angle, with the eye opposite to the batting hand."

In other words, a right-handed, left-eyed batter apparently gets a better view of the approaching pitch than a right-handed, right-eyed batter. The council study said that the latter could overcome his disadvantage somewhat by "opening his stance"—that is, by slightly facing the pitcher instead of standing sideways to him.

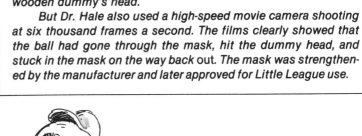

WHAT THE EYES MISS

Some things in sports happen so fast that the eyes cannot follow. Or the eyes and brain don't coordinate quickly enough to interpret the action correctly. Television viewers have the advantage of instant replay, but athletes in the heat of competition don't.

Here's an incident that proves we can't always trust what our eyes tell us:

Some years ago the Little League research director, Dr. Creighton Hale, tested a new plastic catcher's mask, firing a baseball at it from a gun at 120 miles per hour. The ball appeared to stick in the mask, without penetrating far enough to hit the wooden dummy's head.

But Dr. Hale also used a high-speed movie camera shooting at six thousand frames a second. The films clearly showed that the ball had gone through the mask, hit the dummy head, and stuck in the mask on the way back out. The mask was strengthened by the manufacturer and later approved for Little League use.

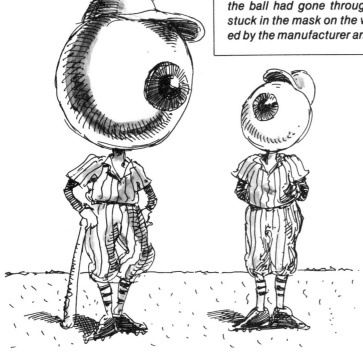

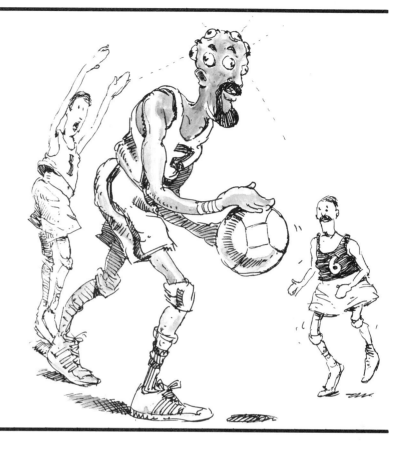

From Tunnel Vision to Cinemascope

Basketball coaches are fond of talking about *peripheral vision*, the ability of a person to see not only what's ahead but also what's on either side. In the case of great passers in sports such as basketball, ice hockey, and lacrosse, it sometimes seems as if they have wide-angle vision—sets of eyes manufactured by Cinemascope.

Former UCLA basketball coach John Wooden says that perhaps those players who don't pass well (or often) "have tunnel vision of their own making." In other words, they want to shoot the goal themselves, and their failure to pass the ball has nothing to do with poor peripheral vision.

Dr. Kenneth R. Diddie, a retina specialist at USC, says there is not much difference in the peripheral vision of healthy people. If one player is a superb passer, Dr. Diddie speculates that it is probably because that player's brain sorts information faster than others.

The Estelle Doheny Foundation in Los Angeles, affiliated with the USC School of Medicine, has an expensive machine called the Octopus, for testing *visual field*—"the area a person can see with each eye when it is fixed on a central spot." While the subject sits with his or her head locked in position, lights flash from all sides. The subject punches buttons if he or she can see blinking lights, indicating where he or she has a normal visual field.

It would be interesting to have such fine passers as Ralph Jackson of UCLA and Earvin Johnson of the Los Angeles Lakers sit in the Octopus' embrace and show off the eyes in the backs of their heads.

Beware the Sun

An athlete outdoors on a sunny day might have to squint to reduce the amount of light reaching his eyes, and squinting can cause fatigue. Glare (bright, dazzling light) can cause errors and accidents: cross-country skiers temporarily blinded by glare can miss the trail, and an outfielder can "lose the ball in the sun." For these reasons, optometrists and oculists recommend wearing sunglasses, which cut down on light and also filter out harmful ultraviolet and infrared rays. Sunglasses should not be worn indoors or at night, as they will temporarily impair the vision and may cause the eyes to become oversensitive to light. But wearing them during the day and then doffing them will help you see better after dark.

Protecting eyes from sunlight is not new. The Chinese wore tinted lenses fourteen centuries ago, according to James Gregg in *The Sportsman's Eye*. Eskimos, faced with bright light reflected off snow and ice, devised goggles made of wood and held on with leather straps.

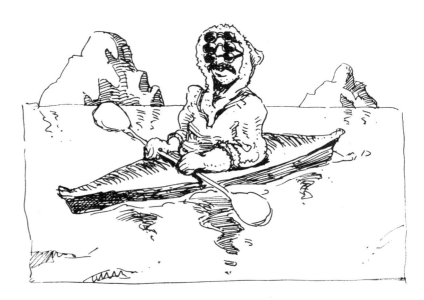

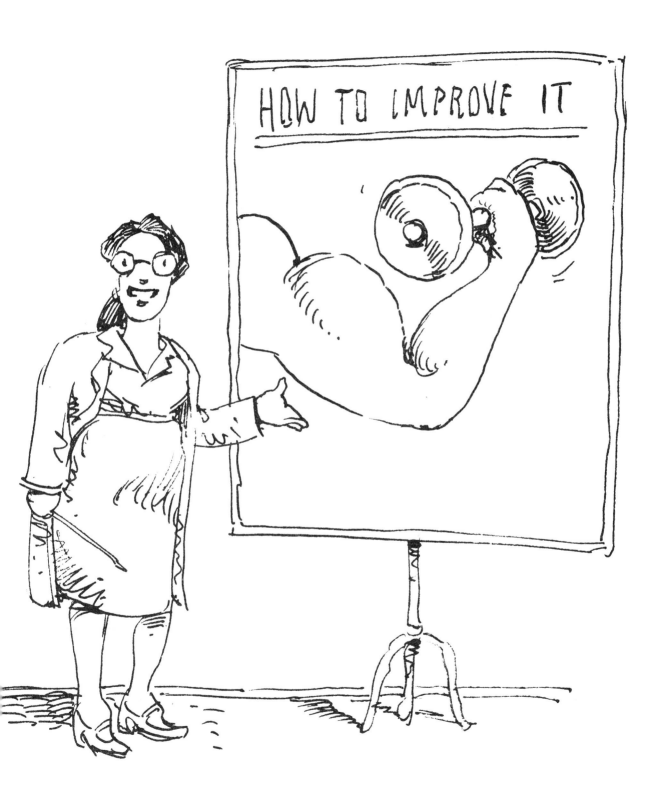

Introduction: Getting the Most from Your Training Time

Knowing how the body works is valuable, but to be successful the athlete usually must know how to make it work *better*. This section concentrates on five possible areas of improvement: strength, muscular endurance, cardiovascular endurance, flexibility, and reaction time and quickness. (Each sport, of course, has a sixth area: technique, or the way skills are used.)

Pole vaulters need strength for planting the pole and pulling themselves up over the bar. But they also need a gymnast's flexibility when their fiberglass poles snap them skyward, and they need muscular endurance to sprint down the runway balancing the pole. Most sports or events are like this, requiring combinations of attributes.

Boxing is one of the few sports that requires all the physical pluses. So when the fine heavyweight from Pennsylvania, Larry Holmes, is training for a fifteen-round title bout—a possible forty-five minutes of continuous punching, blocking punches, and foot-work—he must try to improve all his physical capabilities.

What should be in *your* workouts—stretching, weightlifting, running, standing on your head? Not many sports demand all the attributes. So unless you're set on being a boxer or a competitor in the decathlon (that ten-event ordeal that captures our imaginations at every Olympics), you'll want to use your valuable training time to do what makes you better in your chosen sport.

For example, competitive weightlifting demands strength, flexibility, and technique, whereas marathon running calls for muscular and cardiovascular endurance. The training powerlifter should not waste time developing cardiovascular endurance, and the runner shouldn't bother to develop bulging muscles like Mr. Universe.

Different sports also use these physical attributes in varying ways. Let's take strength as an example. Should it be developed in the legs, arms, hands, chest? A gymnast doing tricks on the parallel bars needs extra upper-body strength. A basketball player needs strong, springy legs for jumping. A shot putter needs *four* strong limbs.

This variety is true of all the pluses: a soccer player must be fleet of foot but not of hand, a basketball player must be both, a skier needs muscular endurance in the legs and the boxer needs it in both legs and arms.

Decide which pluses are needed for success in your sport, then concentrate on the appropriate essay in "How to Improve It" to help organize your training time.

Improving Strength

Records Are Made to Be Broken

It is impossible to predict the limits of human potential in sports (or anything else). Little girls are setting down their dollies at poolside, plunging in, and swimming times that would have won Olympic gold medals in men's competition in years gone by. Athletes, aided by superior equipment (such as the fiberglass vaulting pole), superior coaching, and superior training methods, are getting better in every way: strength, speed, quickness, intelligence.

But in the February 1935 issue of *The Amateur Athlete*, University of California track coach Brutus Hamilton tried his hand at predicting the ultimate marks in his sport. In Table 1 you can see how cloudy or clear his crystal ball was. And Table 2 demonstrates that even for that most glamorous and hotly pursued track-and-field record, the one-mile run, the ultimate in human potential may not have been approached as yet.

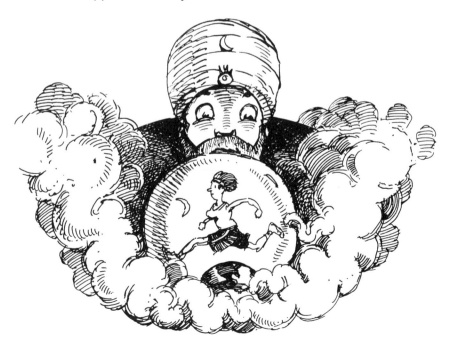

TABLE 1

Progress of World Track Records Beyond 1935 Predictions

Event	The Amateur Athlete February 1935 Predicted Ultimate	Track & Field News January 1981 World Record
Shot put	57'5"	72'8"
Javelin	256'10"	317'4"
High jump	6'11"	7'8¾"
Discus	182'1"	233'5"
Hammer throw	200'3"	268'4"
Pole vault	15'1"	18'11½"
Long jump	27'4"	29'2½"
Triple jump	54'8"	58'8¼"
100 meters	10.6	9.95
200 meters	20.5	19.72
400 meters	46.2	43.86
800 meters	1:46.2	1:42.33
110-meter hurdles	13.8	13.00
400-meter hurdles	50.4	47.13
1,500 meters	3:44.8	3:31.6
3,000 meters	8:05.9	7:32.1
5,000 meters	14:2.36$_{00}$	13:08.4
10,000 meters	29:17.7	27:22.4

TABLE 2

Progress of the World Mile Record

Date	Record-Setter	Time
1875	Walter Slade	4:24.5
1884	Walter George	4:18.4
1895	Thomas Conneff	4:15.6
1915	Norman Taber	4:12.6
1923	Paavo Nurmi	4:10.4
1934	Glenn Cunningham	4:06.7
1937	Sydney Wooderson	4:06.4
1945	Gunder Haegg	4:01.3
1954	Roger Bannister	3:59.4
1954	John Landy	3:57.9
1958	Ron Delaney	3:57.5

Date	Record-Setter	Time
1958	Herb Elliott	3:54.5
1962	Peter Snell	3:54.4
1965	Michel Jazy	3:53.6
1967	Jim Ryun	3:51.1
1975	Filbert Bayi	3:51.0
1975	John Walker	3:49.4
1979	Sebastian Coe	3:49.0

What Is Strength?

Such terms as "strong runner," "strong finisher," and "strong man" blur the distinction between muscular strength and muscular endurance. Intelligent training for sports requires that the distinction be understood.

Muscular *strength* is the greatest force the muscles can produce in a single effort. Imagine discus thrower Mac Wilkins spinning his body and hurling the heavy platter. The distance he throws it is a measure of his muscular strength. The same principle holds true for the shot putter, weightlifter, batter, or high jumper. The force of a single maximum push, heave, swing, or jump is the measure of the performer's muscular strength.

Muscular *endurance* is the muscle's ability to perform many repetitions of the same movement. For example, a sprinter needs muscular endurance to keep those leg muscles churning for fifty or sixty or a hundred yards. (*Muscular* endurance, which is a major requisite for continuous-action sports of all kinds, should not be confused with *cardiovascular* endurance, which comes into play primarily in the long-distance/long-duration events more commonly thought of as "endurance sports." Both forms of endurance will be discussed in detail later on in this book.)

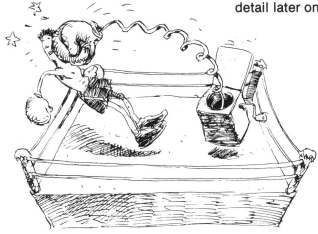

Few sports require *only* muscular strength *or* muscular endurance. Nearly all require both. Brazilian soccer star Pelé, who played in the U.S. pro league for several years, relied on muscular endurance to run the length of the field on attack (a sustained demand on his muscles) and muscular strength to leap up for a head shot in front of the goal (a single explosive effort).

Most sports and events fall between the extremes of discus throwing and running. Figuring out the proper balance between muscular strength and muscular endurance can be difficult. Each athlete must examine each skill used in his sport and decide if it relies mainly on strength or endurance—and to what degree. When in doubt, train for both; no event has ever been lost because the athlete was too well conditioned.

The following essays give advice on improving muscular strength. They are followed by a section dealing with muscular endurance.

Progressive Resistance Training: The Five Principles

Strength training has been practiced for thousands of years. Milo of Crotona, an Olympic-champion wrestler of ancient times (the sixth century B.C.), was a strength trainer. Each day—so the story goes—he lifted his pet baby bull. As the bull matured, gained weight, and presumably got meaner, Milo kept lifting him daily and getting stronger. His system is known today as progressive resistance training (PRT), still the best system there is (not only for developing strength, but for muscular and cardiovascular endurance training as well).

The only difference between PRT and modern variations is the equipment used. Now we have barbells and fancy machines, which are much easier to manage than a raging bull.

PRT can be summed up in five principles of great practical value to athletes.

PRINCIPLE 1: Strength training involves performing a normal body motion while adding resistance to that motion.

A normal body motion is one the body is designed to do. Raise your hand above your head as if reaching for a granola bar on a high shelf, then lower your hand to your shoulder—a normal body motion.

Now put something in your hand (a rock, a quart of milk, your Uncle Max if he's small enough) and repeat the movement. You've added resistance.

PRINCIPLE 2: The strength training program must overload the muscles.

Muscles become stronger or weaker in response to the demands placed on them. If no demands are placed on the muscle, it weakens. (When a person who has been bedridden for a week with Hong Kong flu finally gets out of bed, his legs feel weak. And they are. His muscles have lost strength through disuse.) Overloading the muscle—making a demand close to its capacity—will make it stronger. The strength trainee must overload the muscle to ensure the fastest strength gains. Consider the athlete who can lift a hundred pounds only with a struggle. If he continues this near-capacity lift, his muscles will respond by getting stronger through the creatine/myosin cycle described earlier in "What Makes a Muscle Grow?" Soon the trainee will be able to lift 110 pounds. (If he hefts only fifty pounds, his muscles will not respond; there's no need for them to do so.)

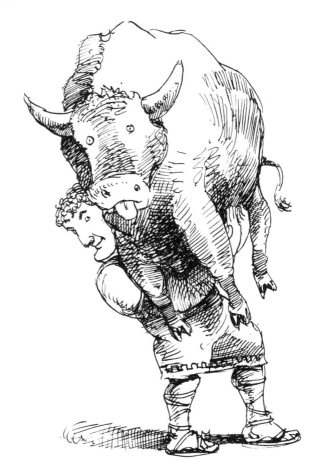

PRINCIPLE 3: As the muscles increase in strength, the resistance must be continually increased.

This principle requires adding weight to the barbell or machine. When lifting ability jumps from 100 to 110 pounds, the trainee must use 110 pounds as his base. By the time this new weight becomes manageable, his strength has again increased and he should jump to 120 pounds. The weight must continue to be increased to keep the gains coming. It changes to 130, then 140 and 150—up, up, up.

PRINCIPLE 4: Strength gains come most quickly with few repetitions and heavy resistance.

Most studies indicate that the greatest strength gains are achieved through three to five sets of two to six repetitions. A set is a given number of repetitions of the same movement with no pause between the movements. Performing more than six repetitions at one time begins to affect endurance rather than pure strength.

The following is an example of a training program designed to improve a basketball player's vertical jump by performing sets of squats using barbells over the shoulders for resistance.

Set number one	6 repetitions
Set number two	4 repetitions
Set number three	2 repetitions
Set number four	2 repetitions
Set number five	4 repetitions

The five sets are done during one training session with three to five minutes rest between sets.

The weight selected for each set should be the most the athlete is capable of handling for that number of repetitions. Anything less will not place maximum demands on the muscles, which is the only way to achieve maximum strength gains. For example, if the basketball player is *able* to do six repetitions with three hundred pounds, he gains no strength by performing fewer repetitions with that weight. Strength gains are achieved only by pushing yourself to the maximum.

PRINCIPLE 5: The muscles must be allowed time to recuperate from the demands of training.

Between training sessions, muscles need rest or they will lose rather than gain strength. The muscles use the recuperative time to replenish energy reserves and mend or build tissue. Thus, most serious weight trainers work on the same muscle group no more than three days a week, usually every other day (with one extra day off between two sessions). So be safe: start with a three-day-a-week training schedule. Later, if you find that's not enough, you can always do more.

Hefting Barbells: Tried and True

Isotonic training has been the mainstay of strength building for three generations. But chances are that if you walked into a gym and said, "Let's train isotonically tonight," you'd get more puzzled looks than workout partners.

Isotonics merely means the use of barbells to develop strength. And barbell training is the most popular form of resistance today. You can find barbells in garages, basements, or school weightrooms around the world. When Walt Frazier was starring on the New York Knickerbockers' first world-championship basketball team, he kept a set in the hotel room he called home.

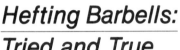

Barbell training has the advantage of economy (an entire set costs about $200) and space (the equipment can easily be shoved under a bed or to the side of a garage). But the greatest advantage is the freedom of movement barbells offer. There's no machine to restrict the body's range of motion.

Any athletic motion can be duplicated with the added resistance of a barbell or dumbbell attached to some part of the body. At your local bookstore there should be books describing the multitude of barbell movements. A good one is *The Gold's Gym Book of Strength Training for Athletes*. Of course, many of you already have a sequence of exercises that you follow. In that case, use your exercises in conjunction with the principles explained in the previous article.

Pushing and Pulling Your Way to Power

When you push against a two-ton truck, nothing moves. But if you push hard enough you feel stress on your muscles. Pushing against any immovable object—wall, door, isometric rack, Notre Dame defensive tackle—creates resistance for the muscles (pushes, pulls, or twists all have the same effect). This immovable resistance is the basis of isometric training. Like weight training, it works by overloading the muscles, but you use no weights or machines.

Isometrics have been around for a long time. During the 1950s, they were billed as the quickest and easiest way to gain strength. Although studies haven't backed up those early claims, it is agreed that isometrics are at least one of the best, quickest, and cheapest ways to increase strength significantly.

When using an isometric training program, follow this advice:

1. Each exercise should be practiced at several joint angles. For example, when doing isometric curls (see Fig. 1), perform a contraction with the arms nearly straight down at the sides; a contraction with the elbows bent at ninety degrees; and a contraction with the elbows bent nearly to the point where the hand meets the shoulder. It's necessary to vary the angle because strength increases are greatest at the angle being trained. Training at many angles distributes the strength gains throughout the range of the muscle's movement.

2. Each muscle contraction (push or pull) should be an all-out, maximum contraction. You must push or pull as

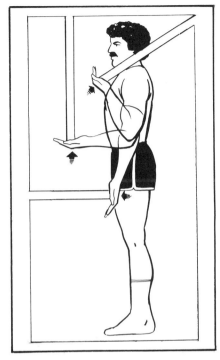

Fig. 1. *Isometric curls performed at different joint angles.*

hard as possible. Remember that you must overload the muscles to induce strength improvement.

3. Each hard-as-you-can push or pull should be held for approximately four to five seconds. Holding the contractions longer than five seconds adds no strength but does cause soreness and fatigue.

4. The isometric contractions should be practiced twice at each angle.

5. Allow two to three minutes' rest between any attempts at the same or different angles.

6. The quickest strength gains come from practicing isometrics every day. Isometrics deplete the muscle's energy reserves much less than other forms of strength training. Also, recovery time, fatigue, and soreness are reduced.

7. Strength gains achieved through isometrics can be maintained by training only once a week. This is probably the biggest "plus" when considering an isometric training program.

Training less than once a week will lead to strength loss. A complete layoff will result in a 60-percent loss in strength within two months. So, if you think you may have only enough motivation to train once a week, isometrics are your best bet.

Special Machines: The Path of Greatest Resistance

Let's review the "iso's": *Isotonic* training consists of hefting barbells. *Isometric* training is pushing or pulling immovable objects. But the best method of strength building through resistance is *isokinetic* training—using special isokinetic devices.

These wondrous contraptions are like magical barbell sets that increase or decrease resistance according to the lifter's capacity at any given point in a motion. Although isokinetic devices *look* very much like the more common Nautilus or Universal machines, the former are, in fact, the *only* machines that can provide maximum stress at every joint angle.

Isokinetic training has been around longer than that old staple of comic-book ads, Charles Atlas's "Dynamic tension." But you've probably not seen the term used much. That's because most gyms don't have the machines on the premises as yet. But that will change as the advantages of these machines become more widely recognized.

Explaining isokinetic training requires a look back to an earlier essay in this book, where you learned that muscles move bones for motion. The angles at which those bones are bent at the joints determines the muscular force which can be exerted. An example you encounter every day is getting to your feet from a sitting position.

If you're sitting in a chair reading this essay, stand up. How did your body respond? If you're like the rest of humanity, the first few inches off the chair were more difficult than the last few inches before standing erect. Why? Because the muscles of the thigh are stressed correspondingly to the angle of the knee joint—greatest at a 90-degree angle (sitting). Conversely, the thighs are strongest as the knees straighten.

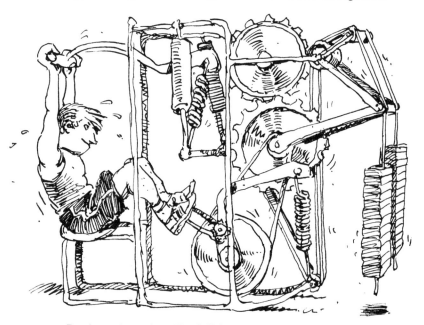

Back to the other "iso's" for a moment. The lack of movement in isometrics means that the same exercise must be done at many joint angles so the muscle is taxed to the utmost through its entire range of motion.

Barbell training (isotonics) has a limited training effect because the maximum usable weight in each movement depends on the weakest joint angle. To understand what this means, imagine our earlier example of standing up from a sitting position. If you want to improve the strength of the movement isotonically, you are limited by the weight you can move the first few inches off the chair (the movement is most difficult at that angle). What's wrong with that? What's wrong is that the weight necessary to add maximum stress to the sitting angle isn't enough to challenge the muscle as the joint nears straightening. Hence, strength at the straighter angle is not improved.

Isokinetic training gives maximum stress on a muscle through a complete range of motion during a single movement, so strength is bolstered at every joint angle. These special machines push back as hard as you push. If you push as hard as you can throughout a movement, the machine gives maximum stress at every angle.

If you're fortunate enough to have access to isokinetic training devices, use them in conjunction with the principles of strength training discussed earlier in this section.

Your Choice of Equipment

The popular, expensive chromed exercise machines made by Nautilus, Universal, and others—so sleek and futuristic that they seem to belong in Darth Vader's arsenal—use the same principles to build muscles as a cheap set of barbells. So the decision on which to use usually boils down to a choice between economy and convenience.

A set of machines costs anywhere from $5,000 to $50,000. A set of barbells that will exercise the same muscles costs less than $200. Modern machines do have the advantage of offering quicker and handier weight selection—an improvement over the sometimes dreary sliding of plates on and off the iron bar. If your wallet is thick enough, perhaps that convenience is worth the enormous cost difference.

Commercial gymnasiums and spas offer elaborate, expensive machines as an added inducement to potential customers. The easier an exercise looks, the more people are tempted to try it, so to some extent the machines are motivational tools.

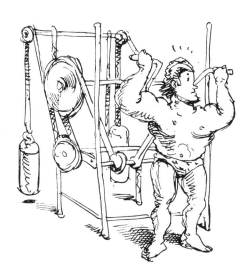
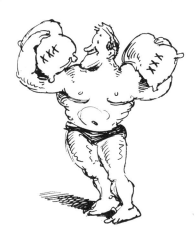

But at the opposite end of the spectrum is the self-motivated high-school tackle exercising in the basement with his trusty set of hand-me-down barbells. He isn't as interested in the conveniences as he is in the results.

Do machines build strength more quickly than barbells? Study after study has said no. The training system and not the equipment determines the rate of strength increase. If you follow the strength-training principles, gains will come as quickly either way. *Effort* spent is the key, not dollars.

It's nice to have machines and barbells to choose from—variety is the spice of training sessions. But you can gain strength by lifting bigger and bigger sacks of sugar. The type of equipment you select is probably the least important decision you'll have to make in planning your program.

Mimic the Movement

If basketball star Earvin (Magic) Johnson wants to improve his jumping ability, he doesn't work on making his neck thicker. You don't have to have a doctorate in physical education to figure out that Magic should exercise his leg muscles. This simple principle is behind the technical term "specificity of movement": improve a movement by strengthening the muscles involved, and do so by mimicking that movement while exercising with weights.

Imagine jumping straight up with a hundred-pound weight strapped to your body. The excess baggage slows your motion and keeps you from really getting off the ground. Then imagine jumping without the extra weight. Your legs straighten more quickly because of the strength/body-weight ratio, and you jump higher. In fact, the faster your muscles straighten your legs, the higher you jump. The difference is the lower resistance without the weight, but the same kind of improvement can come from building up the leg muscles. The stronger they are, the faster they will straighten the legs.

Monitored scientific studies have proven this, with basketball players such as Johnson most often used as test subjects. Players go through a weight-training program to strengthen their thighs and calves—the jumping muscles. Many improve their vertical jumps by as much as ten inches in six months, which means many more rebounds and tip-ins.

The concept of specificity of movement applies to all sports.The shot putter, javelin thrower, quarterback, or polo player should analyze his movements and then approximate them as closely as possible with the weight-training moves.

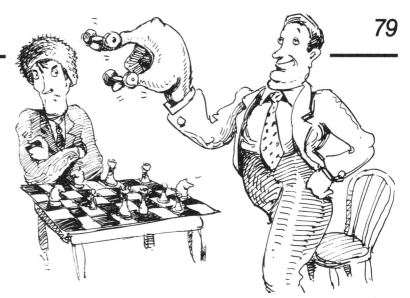

This might mean merely selecting the right muscles to work or changing the angle of a bench to match the angle of release of a shot, ball, or javelin.

Improved strength helps any explosive movement. Boxers, batters, or football linemen punch harder, hit balls farther, or have greater thrust in their blocks. Strengthening all muscles will likely help, but newly developed strength is most effective in those muscles most used in your sport.

A Basic Strength-Building Program for the Entire Body

The basic strength-training program works the major muscle groups. The equipment needed is not elaborate or expensive. A set of barbells or an isometric rack is the basic unit. You'll also need a chinning bar and a set of dip bars, both of which can be built for less than $20.

Two of the four exercises, as shown in Figures 2 and 3, are basic pulling motions (deadlifts and chins) related to movements found throughout sports—pulling an opposing wrestler off balance, rowing, etc. The other two, shown in Figures 4, and 5, are basic pushing motions (squats and dips)—punching, jumping, etc. These four exercises work nearly every muscle in the upper and lower body.

You can supplement the general exercises with specific exercises for your particular sport. To decide the correct number of sets, repetitions, and rate of weight increase when using barbells, refer to the principles of strength training set down earlier in this section.

Two of the four exercises—deadlifts and squats—can be performed isometrically. If you choose this method, refer to the earlier article on isometrics.

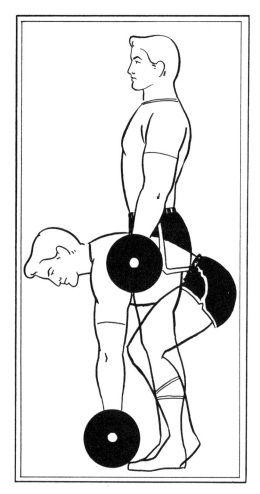

Fig. 2. *As the barbell rests on the floor, bend your knees and grasp it with an overhand grip (palms facing backwards). Keeping your back straight (as opposed to letting it bow), drive with your legs and straighten at the waist until you're standing erect with the bar hanging at arm's length. Return the barbell to the floor. This may be mimicked using an isometric rack or device. Be sure to adjust the rack and repeat for different angles.*

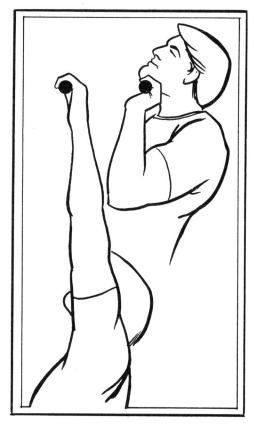

Fig. 3. *With an overhand grip, hang from a bar suspended overhead. Pull your body upward until you touch the bar with your chin. Slowly lower yourself back to the hanging position. As you become stronger, attach a weight to your body as extra resistance.*

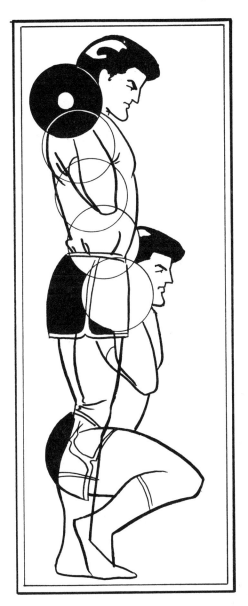

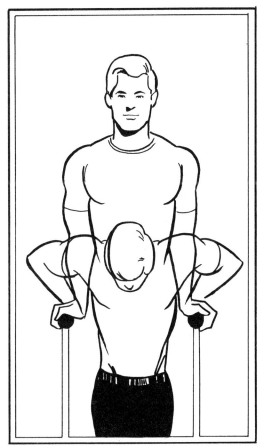

Fig. 5. *Stand between two parallel bars. Grasping them, jump up so that your weight is supported by your hands, with your arms rigidly at your sides. Slowly lower your body by bending your elbows until your upper arms are parallel to the floor. Drive upward using the muscles of your arms, shoulders, and chest until your arms are again straight. As with chins, attach weights to your body as your strength increases.*

Fig. 4. *Place a barbell across the back of your shoulders. From a standing position, bend your legs toward a squatting position until your thighs are parallel to the floor. Drive upward to resume the standing position. This exercise may be mimicked isometrically by adjusting the isometric bar so that your shoulders are pushing against it at various angles of a squatting motion.*

Legs: Building a Good Foundation

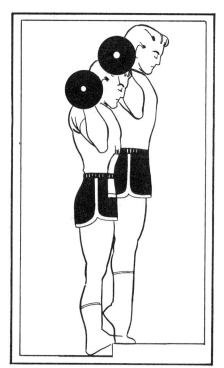

Athletes have long known that their careers end when their legs go. Arrive early at a professional baseball game and you'll see pitchers exercising their legs by running in the outfield, even risking getting skulled by a stray fly ball. The results of laboratory studies show that exercising large muscle groups such as legs and buttocks retards the aging process. Thus, many older athletes lift weights during the off-season to keep their underpinnings strong.

The sprint start, the basketball jump, the glide across the discus circle, and countless other athletic movements involve the legs. Most sports call for complex movements originating with the legs—the jump shot, pitch, swing, and throw, to name a few. That's no surprise when you consider that the legs are powered by the *largest muscle masses* of the human body.

The following is a strength-building program for the legs which should be included in every athletic training program. Strength gains come quickly, since leg-strength potential far exceeds the strength required by normal, everyday demands.

The three exercises in this program were picked as the best of hundreds: leg curls (Fig. 6), calf raises (Fig. 7), and squats (Fig. 8). When doing them, follow the principles of strength training outlined earlier in this section. The principles stay the same regardless of the muscle group being worked.

Remember that all the exercises can be done isometrically. If isometric training is your choice, follow the guidelines discussed in this section.

Fig. 6. *Rise up on the balls of your feet, lifting your heels as high as you can. When you're as high as you can go, lower your heels to the floor again. This exercise can be done either sitting or standing. The resistance can be a bar across your knees if you're sitting or across your shoulders if you're standing.*

Fig. 7. *Lie on your stomach on a bench or floor. Apply resistance to your ankles or feet while bringing the back of your heel toward your buttocks. Lower your foot back into position and repeat. A variation is a one-legged curl in a standing position. For either, use any device such as a Nautilus machine or an "iron boot" that is comfortable and supplies resistance. You can even ask a friend to grasp your ankles and pull on them as you pull in the opposite direction.*

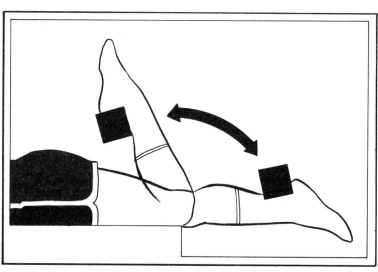

The Steroid Struggle

At the 1964 Olympics, Polish sprinter Ewa Klobukowska was forced to give up her gold medal because tests showed that her hormones weren't normal. At the Montreal Olympics in 1976, six weightlifters (two of them Americans) were ruled ineligible because they had used steroids, which are synthetic derivatives of the male hormone testosterone. In 1979, the International Amateur Athletic Federation banned seven women (three Rumanians, two Bulgarians, and two Soviets) for using steroids.

Steroids have been taken by men in the U.S. at least since 1960, when—wanting to "bulk up" and gain strength—champion weightlifters started gobbling steroid pills like jellybeans. The news soon spread to track-and-field athletes.

One of the early popular steroids was Dianabol, a synthetic hormone clinically used for adding weight to patients debilitated by extended or immobilizing illness. The normal dosage of Dianabol, which is taken in tablet form, was five milligrams per day. Of course, some bodybuilders and other athletes who were willing to make guinea pigs of themselves weren't content with the normal dosage. Many early experimenters took one hundred milligrams daily, and a few tried five hundred milligrams per day!

(That conduct is consistent with what is, in some circles, thought to be a tendency toward addictive personality among competition bodybuilders. In fact, champions in the sport frequently either embrace a zealous, evangelistic religion or turn to drugs or alcohol after their competing days are over. A closer examination might reveal that similar traits are to be found in more than a few intensely competitive athletes in other sports as well.)

Recently, injectable steroids, which are more quickly processed by the human system than tablets, have become increasingly popular. Every year, it seems, more sophisticated injectable steroids are being made available to athletes willing to experiment—Esiclene (Italy), Primabolan Acetate (Germany), and Boleforten (Germany) are three of the latest.

Although there is no question about the strength-building effects of steroid use, an equally important result is water retention in the body, which is responsible for the weight gain that enables bodybuilders to beef themselves up and football linemen to give themselves more padding. The water-retention properties of steroids can cause as much weight gain as *thirty pounds* in three days. Therefore, athletes under the restriction of a weight class must be very careful of steroids. A long program of steroid use in a noncompetitive setting is necessary to ensure the desired results in competitive preparation.

Steroids differ a great deal in their water-retention capabilities: there are steroid combinations that will enhance either strength alone or strength and size together. So a quarterback who wants to gain strength might take one steroid, while an offensive guard who wants to gain both strength *and* size might take another. Even for increasing size, however, water retention has its drawbacks. It can disturb the electrolyte balance in the cells (electrolytes are conductors of electricity), which in turn interferes with muscular efficiency and nerve-impulse transmission.

Furthermore, steroids can affect hormonal balance in serious ways because of the large amounts of male—and sometimes also female—hormones they add to the system. Dianabol, for example, while it improves strength and size, contains a high level of estrogen. This female hormone, in addition to causing a puffy look characteristic of water retention, promotes a mellow, passive and athletically undesirable disposition. And the many steroids that consist primarily of testosterone are said to produce, in women, inappropriately bulky muscles and a degree of aggressiveness beyond the immediate needs of athletic competition.

Other side effects of steroid use are often rumored: deepened voices, facial and chest hair, and menstrual irregularities in women; shrinkage of the testicles, impotency, and stunted growth in men; and possibly liver damage in both. That could be a high price to pay for a blue ribbon or even a big paycheck.

A hue and cry has been raised, with both sides equally intransigent, although the opponents of steroid use seem to have argued their case more vociferously to date—and more successfully too, apparently, since steroid consumption prior to competition has been outlawed by most of the major athletic administrative organizations. However, though rumors have persisted over the years that athletes have dropped dead or incurred grave physical damage from taking steroids, no definitive studies have been conducted to establish a consistent pattern of adverse effects. One thing does seem clear: anyone considering the adoption of a steroid program should investigate the pros and cons thoroughly and proceed only with the utmost caution.

Improving Muscular Endurance

Rapid-Fire Movements

The starter's pistol sounds. Houston McTear bursts out of the starting blocks and sprints one hundred meters to the tape, arms and legs pumping furiously all the way. Sugar Ray Leonard stands in the middle of the ring and slugs it out with his opponent, each of them throwing combinations of punches so rapid that the ringside broadcaster gets tongue-tied. These are examples of *anaerobic* or *muscular-endurance* activities—activities requiring such quick muscle contractions that energy is used faster than the bloodstream can supply oxygen to manufacture it.

Anaerobic activities typically are those lasting from five seconds through one or two minutes that demand quickly repeated, strong muscular contractions. ("Anaerobic" comes from a Greek word that means "without air.") Muscular-endurance or anaerobic events are so named because they differ from *muscular-strength* events (e.g., the shot put), which require one explosive effort at a time, and from *aerobic* or *cardiovascular-endurance* events (e.g., the marathon), which rely on the heart and bloodstream to supply oxygen for the needed energy.

Muscular endurance—as you'll recall from "What Is Strength?"—relies on energy-producing deposits of glycogen already stored within the muscle. But production from these deposits is limited. After one to two minutes of anaerobic effort, the muscle can no longer rely on the glycogen stores for energy (see our earlier article on oxygen debt). At that moment, McTear or any other athlete feels exhaustion, and the muscular contractions slow down to allow the energy deposits to form again.

A Sample Muscular-Endurance Exercise

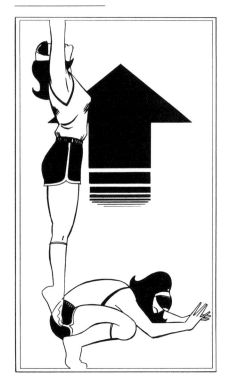

Fig. 9. *This exercise enhances the muscles' capacity to supply energy from their own reserves of stored glycogen.*

Most people learn best through experience rather than reading. So to better understand muscular-endurance training, try the following exercise (designed to improve the endurance of the thigh muscles). Once you've experienced it, the words will mean more.

Start the exercise in a bent-over squatting position as illustrated in Figure 9. Now thrust upward, passing through a standing position, and leave the floor in a jump. Jump as high as you can. As you return to the floor, immediately drop into the squat again. The movement should be quickly up, down, up, down. No pause that refreshes.

Do repetition after repetition as quickly as you can. Make an all-out attempt each time, and be sure to jump as high as possible and drop completely into the squatting position.

Don't feel bad if you last only ten or twenty seconds at first. That's average. In fact, it's unusual for a conditioned athlete—Marcel Dionne or Earl Campbell or Tracy Austin—to last longer than one minute.

Why is this exercise a good example of anaerobic activity?

It relies on *muscular* endurance and not on the cardiovascular system.

The muscle depletes its functional energy reserves because the demand for energy is greater than the speed with which the bloodstream can carry away the poisonous byproducts of energy production.

The aching you feel is caused by lactic acid buildup within the leg muscles.

The panting you experience after completing the exercise is a symptom of oxygen debt. The panting lasts until the lactic acid is eliminated from the muscles.

Stick to Specifics

John Greenshields, a 28-year-old FBI agent, did fourteen thousand sit-ups in a row at the Tampa, Florida, YMCA in 1964. The feat took him six hours, ten minutes. He had practiced by doing a thousand sit-ups before breakfast every day, another five hundred before going to bed, and even more on weekends. Quite a feat. But what was he preparing for? Setting a record, period.

Specificity in muscular-endurance training simply means that the athlete should use the muscles during training as they will be used during competition. Just as important, the training speed, strength, and technique should match the hoped-for competition speed, strength, and technique.

If Greenshields was doing all those sit-ups in preparation for a marathon, his training time was wasted. He should have been working on his legs and cardiovascular system.

A common waste of anaerobic training time is jogging, which lacks specificity and doesn't help the athlete during competition. How many times during a match does a tennis player jog? Never. Jogging is good only for general cardiovascular conditioning, not for muscular endurance.

For an example of the right way to train using specificity, consider a runner preparing to run eight hundred meters in two minutes in competition. During training, he runs four hundred meters in sixty seconds or less, two hundred meters in thirty seconds or less, and one hundred meters in fifteen seconds or less. You can see that each distance is covered at the same pace as that planned for the race—or faster. The muscular demands on the athlete during training match the demands of the race. He will be prepared.

The principle of specificity holds true whether the event be the eight-hundred-meter run, boxing, tennis, or any other muscular-endurance activity. To win, train exactly as you expect to compete.

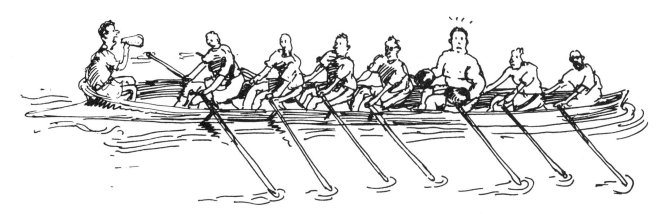

Interval Training for Muscular Endurance

Years of experimentation with various training methods have shown that the best system for developing muscular endurance is interval training: alternate periods of intense anaerobic exercise (work intervals) and rest periods (muscle recovery intervals) in a workout.

The work intervals are short periods of intense, all-out exertions at 90- to 100-percent capacity, which stress the body sufficiently to evoke significant muscular response. They are necessarily short, as it is impossible to move at 100-percent capacity for longer than very brief periods (one to two minutes). And the intensity of the exercise must be at least 90 percent of maximum. Muscular endurance will not be taxed enough with any less effort, and you won't get the desired training effect of forcing the muscles to accommodate ever-increasing stress.

It's easy to figure the magical 90-percent level of capacity for sports that are timed and measured—swimming and track and field. For example, the four-hundred-meter runner capable of a one-minute race will run 360 meters during a one-minute work interval (90 percent of four hundred meters is 360 meters). Calculating a 90-percent effort in wrestling requires the coach and athlete to develop an almost intuitive sense of the athlete's ability. Other coaches, lacking or mistrusting such intuition, demand that the athlete expend a maximum effort during each work interval to make sure that at least 90 percent is reached.

With this type of training, a balance must exist between work and recovery intervals. Recovery must be long enough to allow the muscles to rebuild the energy reserves and eliminate the accumulated lactic acid. So stroll around the gym and admire the calendar art.

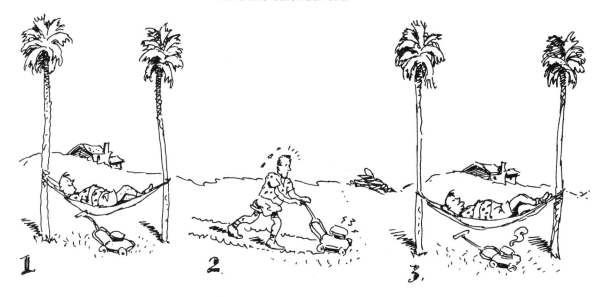

1.   2.   3.

As you might expect, a longer work interval demands a longer recovery interval. A thirty-second work interval requires one to two minutes of recovery, whereas a two-minute work interval might require a recovery interval of fifteen minutes. The longer the work interval, the longer the time needed to eliminate the lactic acid.

Although studies are inconclusive, it appears that interval training sessions should be practiced every other day. (Keep in mind that we are training for muscular endurance and not cardiovascular endurance.)

Here's Howe: Age and Muscular Endurance

Ice-hockey player Gordie Howe played his first minor-league season in 1944–45 and made it to the National Hockey League's Detroit Red Wings in 1946–47. In 1979 he finished his career with the new England Whalers at age fifty-one! That was after 2,106 major-league games and who-knows-how-many scars and bruises.

Muscular Methuselahs such as Howe are rare, of course —especially on skates. One reason is that, like maximum muscular *strength*, the capacity for maximum muscular *endurance* (anaerobic endurance) builds to a peak at about age thirty and then declines irreversibly. The forty-year-old athlete typically has 80 percent of the muscular endurance *potential* he had at age thirty; the fifty-year-old has only 60 percent.

The difference in potential means that the thirty-year-old athlete will develop more muscular endurance than the forty-year-old if both follow the same training program. Mr. Rookie, age eighteen, has about the same muscular endurance potential as Mr. Veteran, age forty, but Rookie's potential increases each year as he heads toward thirty, while Veteran's potential diminishes.

Potential and results don't always follow, though, as Howe showed. Many older athletes are able to beat out younger rivals because they train harder or because of their superior experience or intelligence.

Muscular Strength and Muscular Endurance: Don't Run Out of Gas

Earlier, we carefully examined the distinction between muscular strength and muscular endurance. Now we've come full circle to look at the important connection between the two attributes.

Do stronger athletes have greater muscular endurance —the ability to perform repetitions of a strength movement in rapid succession? Yes, assuming that all other conditioning factors are equal. Hurdler Edwin Moses or rowers on the Harvard crew can use a smaller proportion of their total strength (and thus less effort) to create the same thrust as their weaker opponents. This leaves more fuel in the muscular tank for the stronger athletes, so they run out of gas less quickly.

For example, let's say Bob can manage to do a single curling movement with one hundred pounds, while Joe can curl once with fifty pounds. If both men use twenty-five pounds, Bob will be able to perform twice as many curls as Joe. The strength has given Bob an advantage in muscular endurance.

The muscular strength-endurance connection is one of the reasons males have an advantage over females in athletic competition. Because males can develop greater strength, it follows that they can achieve greater muscular endurance. (Note that we *are* talking about muscular endurance; cardiovascular endurance is another matter altogether.)

To prove the connection we're referring to, find a friend who is substantially stronger or weaker than you are. Using a bag of potatoes, sugar, or other weights, begin lifting. The weight should be approximately half the maximum single-lift capacity of the weaker person. Both of you should curl the weights in rapid cadence. Which of you can curl the weight more times? The stronger person has the greater muscular endurance.

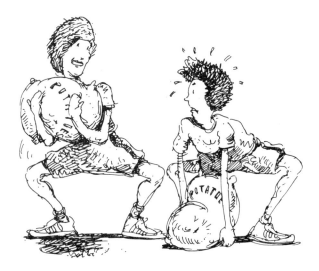

Improving Cardiovascular Endurance

A Cardiovascular Cure -All?

Joggers are clogging the streets, highways, running tracks, and public parks these days. On a snowy day in New York City, a traveling businessman might get in his daily mileage by jogging around an eighteenth-floor hotel hallway in his fashionable sweatsuit. Golfers must watch out for runners using the perimeters of courses. Many people are convinced they are jogging to live longer—running to

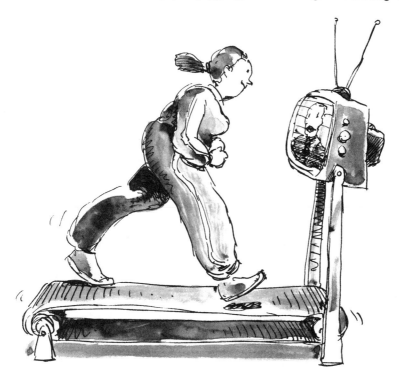

keep appointments with their great-grandchildren, so to speak. And they're right.

The joggers are improving the capacity and endurance of their cardiovascular systems through a program of exercise known as *aerobic training* (a term first popularized in this context by Dr. Kenneth Cooper). Books and articles on aerobic training fill library shelves, newspapers, and magazines. Usually extolling jogging, walking, rope jumping, or swimming, they have a common theme of "improved cardiovascular fitness" through aerobic activities. That is an excellent primary goal for the average person, but only an ancillary benefit for the competitive athlete.

The athlete's main goal through aerobic training: to increase the body's ability to produce new energy. A trained muscle can feed on itself for energy for about two minutes. But for longer periods of exertion, the muscle must rely on oxygen sent by the heart and lungs, delivered via the blood, and "burned" within the muscle. (Remember that *anaerobic* means, roughly, "without air"; conversely, *aerobic* can be defined as "with air"—or oxygen.)

With the goal of improved energy production and access kept in mind, a training routine can be mapped out. As with all other forms of exercise, the basic tenet is progressive resistance training (PRT), or the systematic increase of stress—*over*stress—on the body components being developed. In this case, applying progressively greater demands on the muscles' energy-production capacity—via the heart muscles, lungs, vessels, enzyme production—will force the body to accommodate.

After the body adapts to the first round of demands, more demands must be made so that improvement continues. It's a series of levels, each new one more difficult to reach than the one before.

Jogging relies on this principle. Although the jogger's goal is general fitness rather than competitive athletic performance, the method for accomplishing the goal is the same.

Let's use a hypothetical example, a beginning jogger named Sedentary Sam whose physical activities are pretty much limited to watching TV or walking to the refrigerator to get another piece of cake. Determined to get himself in shape, he spends his first few training sessions walking at a brisk pace (nowhere near the kitchen). As his body adapts to handle these increased demands, he adds a little jogging. Not much at first—maybe only half a mile out of a combined distance of two miles walking and jogging—but an obvious increase over what he's used to. Again the body adapts. Again and again the mileage increases and the body adapts. Sam becomes a budding marathoner. This is not fiction. It frequently happens, as evidenced by modern marathons with more than fifteen thousand entries.

But aerobic events aren't limited to jogging or running. Basketball, boxing, rowing, and soccer, to name a few, require extended periods of intense exercise. Hence aerobic training is a necessity for any sports event lasting longer than our muscles' two minutes of stored energy.

Do you always aerobically train by running, regardless of sport? No. While running is sure to improve the delivery system needed to supply oxygen to the muscles, it doesn't guarantee that any muscle other than the running muscles will effectively use the oxygen. So, unless you're a runner exclusively, use jogging or running only as a supplement.

How do you place aerobic demands on muscles used in a particular sport? By multiple repetitions of the movements used in that sport (applied with PRT). The technique is analogous to that used by our hypothetical Sedentary Sam.

For example, if your sport is boxing, you begin training by punching the bag for three minutes—perhaps at a cadence of one punch every three seconds. Maybe you'll spar for thirty seconds—no easy task for a beginner. As your body adapts to these increased, unaccustomed demands, the demands are

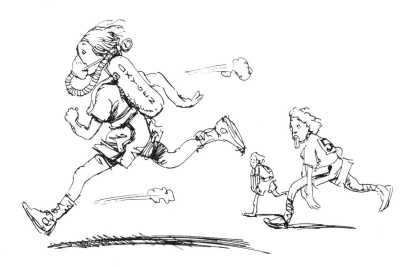

again increased. This time you spend several consecutive rounds on the bag with a punching cadence of one per second. The body accommodates. Again the demands increase; again the accommodation. The particular muscles of your sport are being aerobically conditioned. The use and delivery systems combine to enhance performance.

Whichever of the aerobic-related sports happens to be yours, the fundamentals remain: training time is best spent by placing progressively greater demands on the muscles' ability to produce energy through the use of oxygen. And the basic method of accomplishing this task is to practice the exact movements of your sport.

Improving Flexibility

Flexibility: Sporting Without Strained Muscles

Think of Nadia Comaneci doing a back walkover on the balance beam. Or Pete Rose, prepared to step forward and swing his bat, instead having to duck a high inside pitch. Flexibility in sports means that the athlete has achieved full range of motion in the muscles (full extension and contraction) and a lengthening and increased resiliency of connective tissue in the tendons.

Flexibility is a part of athletic performance that is often taken for granted. Carried away by enthusiasm and a desire to do well, we try things our bodies aren't prepared for: making that sudden change of direction to tackle the tailback, frantically diving to catch a sinking line drive. However, if our muscles are inflexible and weak, we'll be painfully reminded that we should have done some preparing.

Performing flexibility exercises actually lengthens the

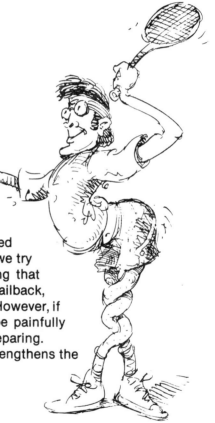

muscles and makes them less likely to tear or pull at the connections with their tendons during movement in the game. A short, inflexible muscle can be easily injured during sudden, jerky movements.

Including a routine of flexibility exercises in your training program can prevent many muscle injuries. Hamstring pulls (at the back of the thigh) are attributed to lack of flexibility of the thigh muscles, which are connected to both the thigh and pelvis bones. Professional football trainers have their players do intensive flexibility exercises daily to keep the leg muscles stretched and pliable; some players are even able to do ballet splits!

Not only do flexibility exercises help prevent muscle soreness and injury, but they can also improve athletic performance. For example, skiers, by flexing the hip rotators and leg muscles during training, can prevent spills on the slopes and enhance their agility and rhythm. For the golfer, flexibility of the torso will ensure full range of motion of the muscles needed for the golf swing. He or she will get more extension on the backswing and in the follow-through.

In determining the flexibility program for your sport, consider which muscle groups are most stressed during competition. Which movements occur most often—reach, turn, bend? The flexibility exercises should stretch those muscles most strenuously used in your sport.

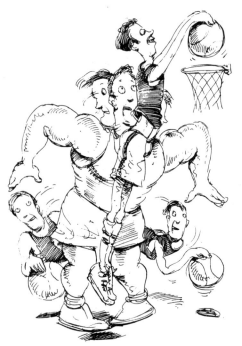

MUSCLE-BOUND BASKETBALL PLAYERS

Basketball is a sport that demands not only agility and flexibility but a fine, delicate shooting touch. Since that touch can easily get thrown out of kilter, many players avoid any kind of exercise that they think will make them "tight" or muscle-bound.

Walt Frazier, the former star for Southern Illinois University and the New York Knickerbockers, didn't believe those theories and worked hard lifting weights and doing isometric exercises. He became an All-American, most valuable player in the National Invitational Tournament in Madison Square Garden, and an All-Pro.

Even his college coach, Jack Hartman (now at Kansas State), thought Frazier was overdoing it one summer in the SIU weight room. "Clyde," as he was later nicknamed, would spend hours going through a routine set up for him by a physical education professor. The next fall, Hartman was surprised at Frazier's improvement—he was much stronger, yet shot as well as ever.

> *Kentucky basketball coach Joe Hall isn't afraid of weight training either. Before the 1980–81 season started, four members of the Wildcat varsity made the Honor Board in the school's weight room for having lifted three hundred pounds in the clean-and-jerk. And the school said seven-footer Sam Bowie had increased his weight from 213 pounds to 237. Others had similar increases.*
>
> *"Most of that is through working on weights," said Hall. "It's good weight—usable, beneficial—not accumulated fat from over the summer."*

Warm Up to Win

Here's a practically guaranteed program for getting beaten, getting injured, or both. Get dressed for your sport—let's say it's volleyball—and walk out on the court just in time for the match to begin. The first serve sails over the net, and you begin digging, blocking, passing, and spiking. If you don't hurt yourself, you're liable to be so far behind by the time you're warmed up that you'll never catch up.

Most athletes have learned that warm-ups improve performance. The muscles perform more efficiently when warmed. During warm-up, as body heat increases:

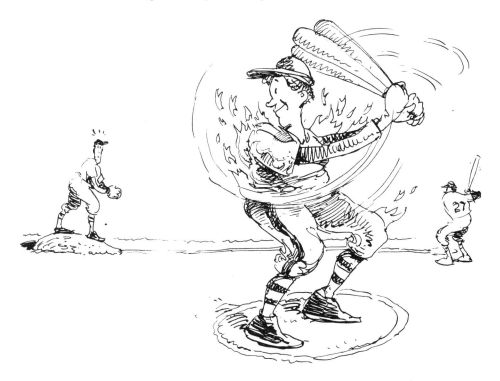

Muscles can contract faster and with more force.

Ligaments and tendons become more pliable.

Nerves conduct impulses faster.

The best warm-up duplicates the movement that is to be performed during training or competition, but it's done less strenuously. For example, tennis player Raul Ramirez starts with easy, soft strokes and gradually increases the velocity of his swing. Pitcher Tug McGraw begins by merely lobbing the ball to his catcher.

Some athletes reportedly have used passive warm-up methods such as infrared light application, massage, saunas, and hot showers. Sandy Koufax, the great pitcher for the Los Angeles Dodgers a few years back, had difficulty getting "loose." The team trainer at the time, Wayne Anderson, said Koufax's back was more muscular than any pitcher's he'd seen in eighteen years in the major leagues. Anderson rubbed a hot, red ointment into Sandy's back before each turn on the mound. However, usually these methods offer little value because they fail to significantly raise the muscle temperature.

There is another important reason for warming up by mimicking the movements of the competitive event: to prepare the nerve pathways for an all-out effort. Muscle contractions are activated by nerve impulses, which act with better timing and greater intensity when given a little practice. The muscles contract at the right rate. The throw or lift is straighter or stronger.

General warm-ups such as slow jogs or jumping-jacks do raise muscle temperature, but they don't condition the nerve pathways. Therefore, the athlete should mimic the heavy-training movement with a nonstrenuous movement.

The warm-up also appears to help prevent injuries. Although not verified by controlled studies, the practical experiences of coaches and athletes strongly support the injury-prevention value of warm-ups.

Improving Reaction Time and Quickness

Reaction Time: Getting Out of the Blocks

Sprinter James Sanford is ready in the starting blocks. His race begins with the bang of the starter's pistol. The split seconds between the gunshot (stimulus) and Sanford's first movement (overt response) constitute his reaction time. Let's take a closer look.

The gunshot starts the sequence. The vibrations from that shot reach his ears. Nerve impulses travel from his ears to his brain. His brain must separate the gunshot impulses from others received at

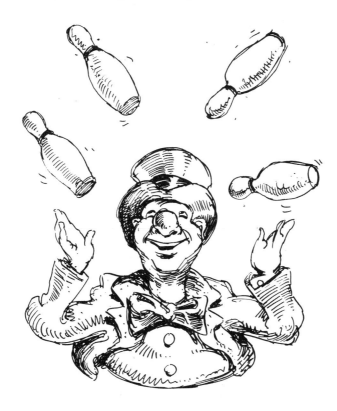

the same instant (crowd noises, a burp from the fellow in the next lane).

After singling out these impulses, his brain decides how to respond. An appropriate message is then sent to those muscles needed to begin that first perceptible movement out of the blocks. And all this happens in the blink of an eye.

The average reaction time to sound is 120 to 180 thousandths of a second—determined under laboratory conditions in which the sound came through headphones and the response was pressing a button. Similar studies indicate that reaction time to visual stimuli was longer—150 to 225 thousandths of a second.

These statistics relate to simple reactions (hear a buzzer, press the button). More complex reactions take more time, and athletic reactions usually are more complex. Keeping in mind the stimulus-brain-muscle sequence, imagine the complications of responding to an opposing table-tennis player's forehand smash.

You can improve reaction time through practice. The brain's ability to differentiate is of prime importance. The more closely the stimuli resemble one another, the longer the reaction time. Practice gives the brain repeated chances to sort out the stimuli and make an appropriate response. In other words, understand the message received and send the appropriate muscles into action. This holds true for every sport.

For example, a beginning boxer learns to defend against an opponent's jab by catching it with his own gloved hand. Repeated practice increases the fighter's ability to do so by shortening the reaction time—the brain more quickly differentiates among a jab, a cross, an uppercut, and a hook.

Reaction time shortens, of course, if the athlete is prepared to react. A simple example is Clancy Edwards, poised and waiting for the starter's gunshot: on your mark, get set, bang! Be prepared for the gunshot, the dropped puck in the faceoff, and so on. Multiple repetitions of every movement allow the brain to pick apart the elements of each stimuli, thereby producing a faster reaction time.

In addition to lack of preparation, fatigue, drugs, alcohol, altitude, and advancing age hinder reaction time. With increasing fatigue, reaction time lengthens because the brain's receptor, integrator, and transmitter cells become unable to process inputs quickly when they body is tired.

Drugs and booze can interfere with the rate at which the brain sorts through stimuli. Consequently, both are taboo for athletes.

The relation between altitude and reaction time is not understood precisely. However, air density (which affects the way sound travels) and unusual gravitational pull are factors now being investigated. Of course, lessened oxygen at higher altitudes could lead to a loss of sorting ability in the brain.

The Hand Is Quicker than the Fly

There are flamboyant athletes—braggarts of the Muhammad Ali type—who claim they are so quick that they cannot only catch a fly in midair, they can catch it between thumb and forefinger. That's quickness, all right—which is different from reaction time.

The quickness of a movement is measured from the stimulus to the completion of a response. Reaction time is measured from the stimulus to the start of the response.

What will improve quickness? Stepping up reaction time will help because it is a component of quickness. Also, improving the speed of the movement itself will improve quickness.

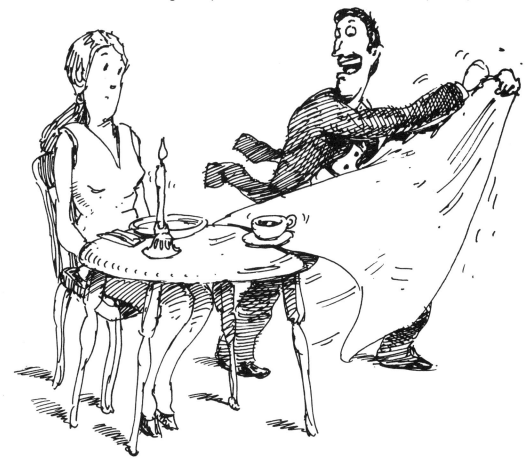

All athletic movements depend on muscles moving bones for motion. Therefore, we need to ask what factor or factors will enhance the muscles' ability to move these bones. The primary factors are practice and strength.

Practice provides preparedness. The brain learns to respond unhesitantly with the appropriate intensity and number of impulses to the muscle. These impulses determine the strength with which a muscle is contracted. And the strength of the contraction determines the speed of movement as the muscle pulls the bone.

Of course, the brain's command doesn't mean much if the muscle is weak. That's the reason the athlete should try to achieve an increase in strength. Study after study concludes that an athlete improves quickness by improving strength. Stronger muscles can make stronger contractions, which in turn pull bones more quickly.

Hence, training for cobra-strike or fly-catching quickness boils down to two ingredients: (1) practice your event for improvement in reaction time and movement, and (2) develop more strength.

Special Conditions

From Altitude to Dimples

The athlete with more talent and better conditioning than his opponents usually wins. But note that word *usually*. Luck, intelligence, and concentration all play a part in competition, and so do special conditions. For example, a great Olympic pole vaulter using an old-fashioned bamboo pole might not be able to beat a good high-school vaulter using a modern fiberglass pole.

Here are a few more examples of special conditions:

ALTITUDE:

At the 1968 Olympic Games in Mexico City, Bob Beamon of the U.S.A. shattered the world long-jump record by more than *two feet* with a leap of 29 feet, 2¼ inches. Many experts considered the jump the greatest feat in track-and-field history. Before that jump, the world record had increased by only six inches in twenty-five years.

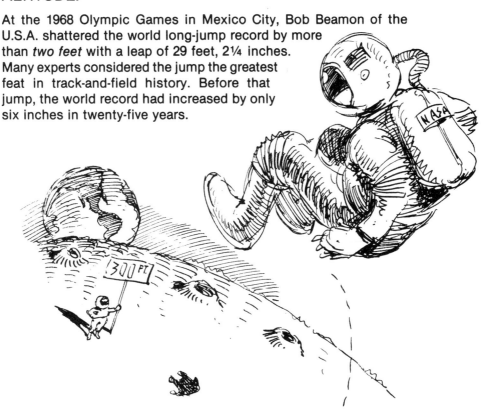

Did the seven-thousand-foot elevation of Mexico City contribute to the amazing distance? Yes! The difference in gravity and air resistance at the higher elevation helped a good jump become a great jump.

The pull of gravity on the body lessens as you get closer to the equator and higher in altitude. But calculations indicate that the weaker pull of gravity on Beamon's body added only 1¼ inches to the jump—certainly not two feet. The density of air at sea level is approximately 1.3 times as great as the density of air at Mexico City. The diminished air resistance on the jumper figures out to an added thirty-one inches of distance!

Subtracting the added distance achieved as a result of competing at Mexico City's altitude, the jump would have measured 26 feet, 6¼ inches at sea level. The astounding world record in Mexico City would have been merely a good jump at most other places.

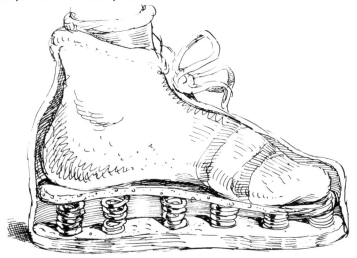

PITCHES AND ATMOSPHERE

Baseballs as well as baseball players respond to weather changes. For example, on cool, dry days, fastballs slow up and curveballs curve more.

The air is heavier and more densely packed on cool, dry days, and the greater the air density, the greater the air resistance to the ball as it moves through the air. That explains why a fastball slows up in densely packed air—it's harder for the ball to move through it. But why does dense air help the curve?

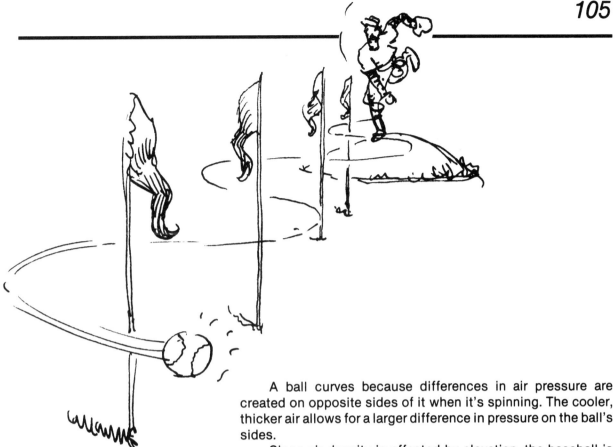

A ball curves because differences in air pressure are created on opposite sides of it when it's spinning. The cooler, thicker air allows for a larger difference in pressure on the ball's sides.

Since air density is affected by elevation, the baseball is affected by differences in altitude. A fastball will be faster in higher, thinner air (Denver's minor-league ballpark, for instance). But the pitcher's advantage over the batter is somewhat offset because a batted ball will travel farther.

SPAGHETTI RACKET

Before this tennis weapon came into prominence in 1977, rules about rackets were practically nonexistent. Dick Stockton and Stan Smith could go out on the court and rally back and forth using Ping-Pong paddles if they wanted to.

Then the controversial Rumanian, Ilie Nastase, and some other tour regulars started using the spaghetti racket, double-strung in such a way as to cause more and crazier spin on the ball. The International Tennis Federation said it threatened the character of the game and outlawed it, which set off a court battle with the manufacturer. The ban was upheld by a U.S. District judge early in 1981.

DIMPLED GOLF BALLS

The earliest golfers used balls made of smooth pieces of leather packed with feathers. Peculiar things happened to those early balls. As they became scuffed and pitted, they traveled farther. This prompted manufacturers to develop dimpled golf balls. How do dimples help the flight of a ball?

A smooth golf ball spins forward, pushing air ahead of it. The pressure at the rear of the ball decreases because less air is present (air does not have time to completely fill in behind the ball as it zooms forward). High air pressure in front and low air pressure in back cause the ball to drop.

Dimples on the ball act as little air pockets, carrying air from the front to the rear. Consequently, the pressure at the rear more closely matches the pressure at the front. The ball sails farther—in fact, about five times farther.

Recently, Polara Enterprises, Inc., introduced a ball with dimples of varying depth and billed it as a straighter flyer—hook-resistant and slice-resistant. The U.S. Golf Association refused to approve it.

The lesson here is: Pay attention not only to your body but to important things around you, including atmosphere and equipment.

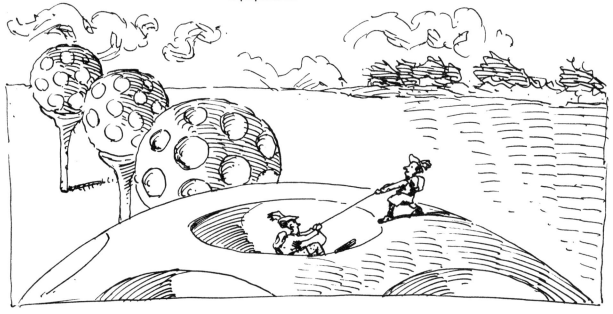

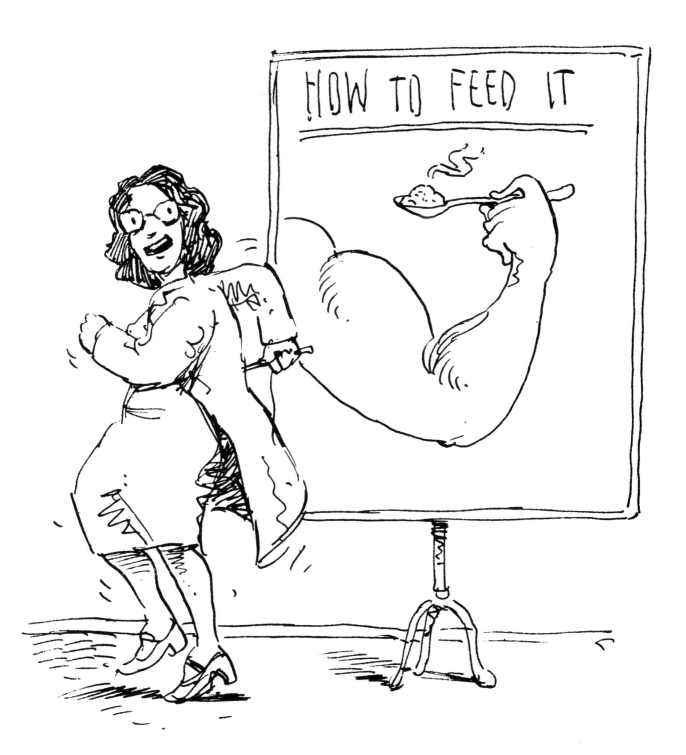

Introduction:
The Athlete's Diet

*T*he saying, "You are what you eat," is true. Of course, that means some people probably have the body chemistry of jelly doughnuts. What you eat also partly defines what you are able to *do*. Papaya juice, Reggie candy bars, *crepes suzette*, Big Mac hamburgers—all food is energy. The athlete's concern is getting enough energy to help him or her score a goal, serve an ace, or paddle a canoe through the rapids. Only the best high-test fuel is pumped into Indianapolis race cars, and it should be no different for otherwise finely tuned human beings.

Foods differ drastically in the amount of energy they supply and the speed with which they supply it. Knowing a particular food's capabilities allows you to plan your meals properly in relation to workouts and competition.

Every person should be careful about diet. In fact, the best diet for an active athlete is not much different than for a sedentary accountant. Training and competition do make some extra demands, which we will discuss in this section. And we'll serve up foods according to their components: protein, fat, carbohydrates, vitamins, minerals, and water. All are not only important but essential to life.

The Athlete's Energy Requirements

Counting Calories

Different characteristics of the athlete's body are measured with different units: height in feet and inches, weight in pounds—familiar, easily understood terms. His energy needs are measured with slightly less familiar units, calories. Most people have heard of calories in connection with diets but know them only as vague units of guilt or something Rocky Road ice cream has a lot of.

A calorie is a measurement of heat energy. Energy comes in other forms, such as light and electricity, but heat is the basis of the calorie. A calorie is about the amount of heat it takes to raise the temperature of a quart of water two degrees (F).

You can capture calories from fire by heating a quart of water in a teapot. Each time the temperature rises two degrees, you've captured one calorie in the water. You can then lose them again by placing the teapot in the freezer. The calories will escape into the

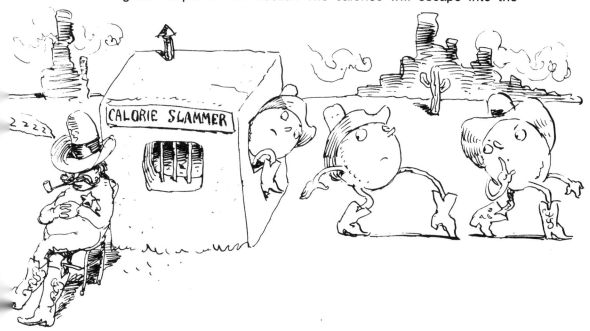

atmosphere as the water cools—one calorie lost for each two-degree drop.

The athlete, like all of us, gets calories (energy) from food. Different foods provide different amounts of energy. A piece of chocolate-cream pie can be converted into hundreds of energy-producing calories, but water provides us with none because the body doesn't know how to convert water into vigor.

In a laboratory, the number of calories available from an apple, an orange, or a piece of pie can be determined by measuring the amount of heat it takes to completely burn them. The food contains one calorie if the heat required to burn it would raise the temperature of a quart of water by two degrees. Eighty calories means that an equivalent amount of heat would raise the temperature of eighty quarts of water two degrees each.

Fortunately, you don't need a lab to check the various calorie contents of food; just get a "calorie counter"—that is, a booklet containing a food-by-food evaluation of calorie content. You can find these for less than a dollar at most supermarkets. It's the easiest way to check.

BMR: Keeping the Body Humming

Metabolism is a word that comes into the conversation when talk turns to the body's need for food energy. "High metabolism" and "low metabolism" are expressions that are tossed about almost as easily as the weather or the time of day. Just what is metabolism?

Scientifically, metabolism can be defined as "all chemical reactions within the body that require energy." Unscientifically, it means the energy needed to perform every heartbeat, gland secretion, muscle twitch, yawn, and thought—in other words, everything.

The body needs energy just to stay alive. The rate at which it uses energy to maintain itself, without any extra physical activity, is called the basal metabolic rate (BMR). The BMR keeps things like the heart, lungs, and glands functioning so you can devote your conscious efforts to screwing in the lightbulb or doing a triple backflip off the diving board. BMR also maintains body weight. The average-sized adult requires about eighteen hundred calories each day to satisfy the energy consumption of the BMR. That requirement differs from person to person because of such things as weight and output of the thyroid gland.

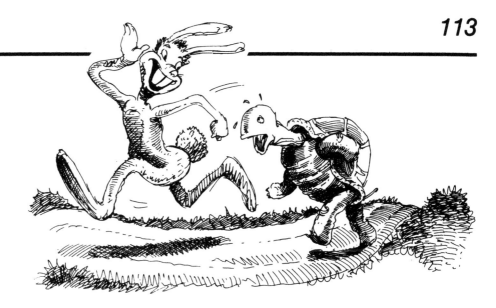

(How does the body know when it needs nourishment? When the stomach is empty, strong, slow muscular contractions of its walls stimulate nerve endings there. The nerve endings, or receptors, in turn send hunger messages to the brain. Scientists haven't figured out all the other sources of hunger signals, but they certainly exist, because people who have had their stomachs removed still have appetites.)

The metabolic rate beyond the BMR depends on the activity level of the particular person. Although thinking does soak up energy, the atomic physicist who sits and theorizes all day *á la* Albert Einstein doesn't need as much as jockey Bill Shoemaker riding in eight races at Santa Anita. It's supply and demand. The more demands placed on the body, the higher the energy expenditure and the higher the metabolism.

It follows that different sports require different energy expenditures and raise the metabolic rate to different levels. The athlete meets the increased energy demands by placing more food in the system. The food energy must balance the energy spent.

Pancakes or Steaks: Energy Contributions of Various Foods

We all know at least one enthusiastic trencherman who never met a calorie he didn't like. But are all calories the same? No. In simple terms, carbohydrates (pancakes, waffles, granola, non-diet cola) are used for both short-term and long-term energy supplies. Fats (bacon, butter) are a long-term energy supply. Proteins (steak, leg of lamb) are a constant growth and repair source and can also be changed in the body to carbohydrates or fat.

Extensive studies to determine the caloric values of carbohydrates, fats, and proteins estimate the amount of energy supplied as:

1 gram of carbohydrate	= 4 calories
1 gram of fat	= 9 calories
1 gram of protein	= 4 calories

(A gram, by the way, is one thousandth of a kilogram, equal to 15,432 grains. Therefore, a gram cracker is much smaller than a graham cracker.)

To set up his or her diet, the athlete must know which source will most quickly supply vigor and vim. The most easily converted and readily available source is the sugars and starches of the carbohydrate group. Although fats are a more concentrated energy source, their conversion to usable energy is more complicated and time-consuming.

Protein is the least efficient energy source to convert because the conversion process is even more difficult than for fats. (In other words, it takes too long for a pork chop to become a knock-out punch.) In general, the body only uses protein for energy when the more efficient carbohydrates and fats aren't available.

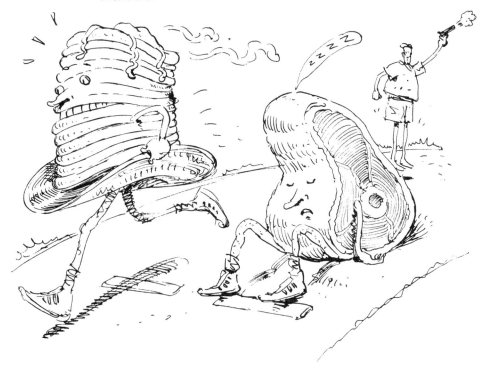

The Basic Nutrients

Introduction:
The Basic Nutrients

All the food we eat—from snails in garlic butter to banana-cream cake, from asparagus in hollandaise sauce to liver and onions—can be broken down into six groups, each of which has special qualities that satisfy different body needs. Water, proteins, fats, carbohydrates, vitamins, and minerals are collectively called the "basic nutrients."

They have three big jobs to do: supply energy, enable tissue to grow and be repaired, and catalyze or otherwise participate in the body's thousands of life-supporting chemical reactions.

These next few articles explain how the body depends on these nutrients.

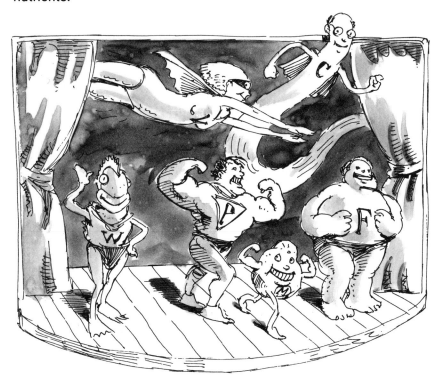

You're All Wet!

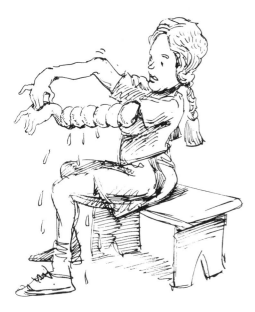

Almost three-fourths of the earth's surface is covered by water. Likewise, about 60 percent of the human body is water. It's a good thing, too, because even though water has no calories, vitamins, minerals, or usable energy, it is second to oxygen as the most immediately needed substance. Without an adequate supply, we would quickly—as it were—kick the bucket.

Most (about two-thirds) of the body's water content is located in the cells, in varying proportions depending on the type of cell. You can think of the cells as containing chemical structures floating in liquid. It's a wonder we don't slosh when we move.

The other large concentration of water is in the blood. The average athlete has about a gallon of water as blood fluid. Floating along in this stream are the oxygen-carrying red blood cells and lots of food, vitamins, and minerals that must be delivered to the cells.

Water is also necessary to the body's cooling, lymphatic, and nervous systems and acts as a safety cushion to the spinal cord, joints, and brain. It's instrumental in every body function.

Humans get water from three general sources. The most obvious is the liquids we drink. But substantial amounts are contained in so-called solid food, too. (The percentages of water run from less than 5 percent in a soda cracker to more than 90 percent in a stalk of celery and a head of lettuce.) The third source is energy metabolism. As carbohydrates, fats, and proteins are metabolized, varying amounts of water are released into the system.

In just a few hours of intense competition in hot weather, an athlete can easily lose 5 percent of his or her body's water. Even the Sedentary Sams and Susies lose substantial amounts through evaporation and urination—so much that they would die in several days without replenishing the supply.

Water should be supplied continually, even during exercise. But gulping down huge amounts at one time won't do anything but bloat the stomach and make you feel as if you've swallowed a watermelon whole. The bloodstream can only absorb about a quart per hour, so the best method is to take small, frequent drinks. When the body is low on water, every system and every cell are affected: the cooling system falters and the body temperature rises; the blood begins to thicken, causing the circulatory system to malfunction; elimination of waste is inhibited; the nervous system goes haywire; and the athlete's strength, coordination, and overall performance break down. Water's cheap. Use it.

Protein Is
No Panacea

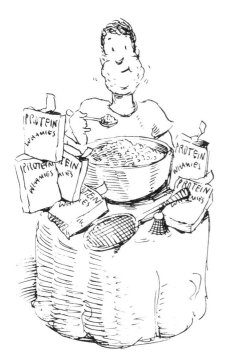

For a long time athletes believed that their bodies needed great quantities of protein. If a breakfast-cereal box advertised its contents as "Rich in protein!" the budding badminton star would hasten to buy. However, up-to-date studies have shown that badminton players probably need no more protein than law clerks or mattress testers—fifty to seventy grams a day for an average-size man (160 pounds).

But protein is nonetheless essential to the body's functioning. Digestion breaks protein down into the basic building blocks, amino acids, which are responsible for the formation, growth, and maintenance of all the body's cells.

Your body needs twenty-two different amino acids for proper maintenance and growth. The body can manufacture fourteen of these from other food eaten in a normal diet. However, the other eight, called the essential amino acids, must be obtained from protein sources on a daily basis, since amino acids are not stored in the liver, lungs, lymph glands, or anywhere else from head to toe.

Raw protein foodstuffs are classified as complete or incomplete. A complete protein is one that has all eight essential amino acids. An incomplete protein is one that lacks one or more of the essentials. Common sources of complete protein are meat, eggs, and milk. Few plants have complete proteins, so don't look for asparagus spears to become building blocks.

Not all the essential amino acids have to come from the same food source. The important thing is that the total food intake supplies the essentials. Peanuts and peas, while not being complete proteins in themselves, combine to supply all eight essential amino acids. Once the amino acids are created in the digestive system and enter the bloodstream, they are all treated the same; the original source doesn't matter.

Lack of enough protein is rare in industrialized countries. Considering that a quart of milk contains thirty-two grams of complete protein, you can see how easy it is to get a day's supply of fifty to seventy grams. Keep in mind, though, that too much protein can cause physical problems by overworking the liver and kidneys.

A Love Note
to Lard

Don't let the word "fat" scare you. You *need* fat in your diet—and hanging (lightly) on your body—to stay healthy and energetic. Be glad you don't have the same sort of energy-storage system as a palm tree, or you'd have to have a liver the size of a coconut.

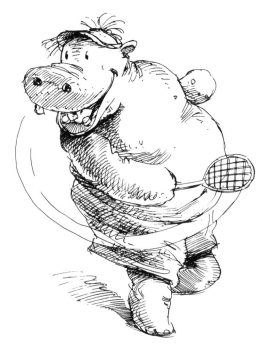

To explain: Plants store energy in the form of carbohydrates, and animals store it in the form of fats. If humans stored all their energy as glycogen (the body's form of carbohydrate storage), it would take twenty pounds to keep two days' worth of energy. The same five thousand calories can be stored in one and a half pounds of body fat!

It's well known that there is lots of fat in butter, margarine, and vegetable oil. But all other foods contain fat, too, varying from less than 1 percent in most fruits and vegetables to 100 percent in lard.

Fats have the highest concentration of energy of all foods—more than forty-two hundred calories per pound, compared to about seventeen hundred for carbohydrates. After becoming part of the body, stored fat has an even greater energy advantage: thirty-five hundred calories can be pulled from a pound of fat compared to 250 from a pound of glycogen stored in the liver. That's a great many more strides, swings, or punches.

Fat is the main source of energy stored in the body. But you don't have to eat it to store it, because both proteins and carbohydrates can be converted into body fat. In fact, nearly everything digested—from cantaloupe to cashew nuts—can be converted and stored as fat. (This can be taken to extremes. The body doesn't have a storage cabinet that's locked when full. The more excess food eaten, the more fat stored and the larger the belt size.)

Fat acts as internal padding, which is vital for protecting organs from impact damage. A kidney or liver could be severely injured during a football game or boxing match if the organ weren't surrounded by a fat cushion. Subcutaneous fat—suet just under the skin—also acts as insulation against the cold.

One final, important need for fats in the diet has to do with their ability to carry vitamins that are not water-soluble—those vitamins that can't ride through the body in water but can in fats. Without fats, these essential nutrients, vitamins A, D, E, and K, could not be absorbed and used by the body.

Stored fat is in constant flux. Each week about half the body's fat is involved in various metabolic processes, and half is replaced. But the relative percentage of fat stays the same unless the balance of calories taken in and calories used is changed.

Since fat foods take longer to convert to energy, it's best that the athlete rely more on carbohydrates as the major energy source. Most sports-medicine specialists recommend that the athlete get about 20 to 25 percent of his or her daily dietary supply from fat. Also, it's not a good idea for the athlete to store any more fat than accounts for 10 percent of body weight. This percentage will allow for an emergency energy supply while keeping the body athletically lean.

Carbohydrates for Quick Energy

Although not as efficiently stored as fats, carbohydrates are the main source of food energy for human beings. Such things as tangerines, dried figs, and French bread are loaded with carbohydrates, which are composed of the starches and sugars found in plants. Chemically speaking, they're complicated mixtures of hydrogen, oxygen, and carbon.

We will attempt to discuss the process by which the body converts carbohydrates into energy—a highly complex subject—as simply as possible in the following paragraphs.

Carbohydrates are divided into three categories that sound like the names of ousted Greek premiers: monosaccharides, disaccharides, and polysaccharides. "Saccharide" essentially means sugar. "Mono," "di," and "poly" indicate the number of sugar molecules in the carbohydrate—meaning one, two, and three or more, respectively.

The body can pass only monosaccharides (single sugar molecules) from the intestine into the bloodstream. Although digestion breaks down most di's and poly's into mono's for use

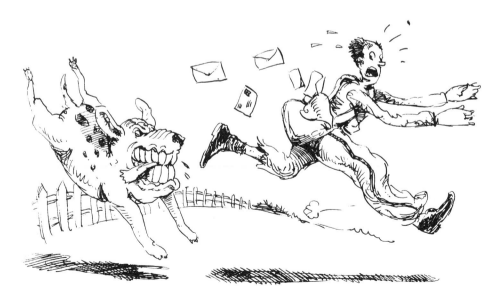

by the body, some strings of sugar molecules are too complex to be thus broken down. These carbohydrates, found in foods such as lettuce and celery, pass through the system as roughage and aren't converted to energy. They're excellent diet foods.

Only three monosaccharides are able to pass from the intestine to the bloodstream: glucose, fructose, and galactose. Glucose is the body's basic energy source because of the ease with which it passes from the intestine through the bloodstream to the area of energy demand. For example, eating a candy bar or a spoonful of honey yields quick energy because both sugar and honey contain natural glucose.

The other two mono's (fructose and galactose) must make a stop at the liver in order to be made over into glucose. This glucose is then sent into the bloodstream to be used where immediately needed. If not needed right away for a sprint or a swim, it is stored in the liver and muscles as glycogen.

Glycogen is needed in two sets of circumstances. The first occurs when not enough carbohydrates have been consumed in foods to supply the body's general energy needs. The liver then releases some glycogen into the bloodstream. The second set of circumstances is familiar to you: during anaerobic activities the glycogen stored within the muscles is used for energy, and it's used at an even greater rate when the bloodstream can't deliver oxygen fast enough.

Carbohydrates must be included in the daily diet, mostly because the body stores less than a pound and that doesn't go very far. For example, during a race the average marathon runner burns more energy than a pound of carbohydrates supplies.

Carbohydrates are much more quickly digested and turned into energy than fats. Likewise, stored carbohydrates (glycogen) can be more quickly tapped for energy than the body's fat supply. But that's OK, because by the time the relatively small amount of stored glycogen is used for an emergency, the greater amount of fat has had a chance to gear up and come to the rescue. They work as a team. One's a fast starter and early finisher, while the other comes in late in the game but keeps the momentum going.

Without a moderate supply of carbohydrates, the muscles can't be properly maintained or trained. That's because carbohydrates regulate protein metabolism; in other words, they must be present to allow the body to assimilate protein for building and repairing the muscles. And the brain depends on the bloodstream's supply of glucose—which is sent there by carbohydrates—for energy, since the brain can't store its own energy.

It's obvious why carbohydrates are an important nutritional element. Considering how easily they are obtained from food, only a fool would go without them. Even the low-carbohydrate diet recommends that the dieter take in sixty grams of carbohydrates a day.

Vitamins for Vitality, But Don't Overdose

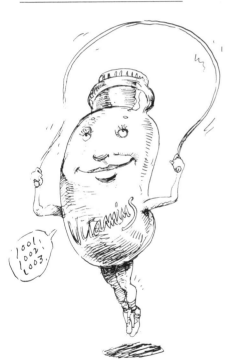

The word *vitamin* comes from the Latin word for life, which is appropriate since those invisible organic substances we call vitamins are so important to our well-being. Trying to function normally on a racquetball court or anywhere else without them would be like trying to run a bakery without flour.

All foods contain vitamins, but no single food has them all, which is why the athlete is constantly reminded to have a well-balanced diet. Vitamins don't directly add structural form or energy to the body's tissues, but they are essential helpers in all the maintenance, building, and energy-producing processes. They play a major role in forming thousands of compounds needed for cell activity. Depriving the body of just one type of vitamin sets off a chain reaction that halts the formation of thousands of these compounds. Vitamins are either fat-soluble or water-soluble. That is, some need to combine with fat in order to carry out their duties and others need to swim, so to speak. Even to make it from the intestine into the bloodstream, they must travel with the proper partner.

Chances are that missing a few days' supply of fat-soluble vitamins (A, D, E, and K) won't hurt you, because those are stored by the body and can be taken out of storage if need be. Excessive quantities of fat-soluble vitamins, particularly in the liver, can create a toxic effect—vitamin poisoning. Lots of well-meaning athletes have done themselves more harm than good by wolfing down vitamin supplements like so many gumdrops. The symptoms are sluggishness and indigestion, which aren't likely to help you field a hard-hit ground ball or sink a putt.

Water-soluble vitamins aren't stored—take too many, and they're washed out with the urine. But without a daily supply of what *is* needed, the athlete's performance is hurt. For instance, not enough B-complex lowers the speed of nerve impulses and produces cramps, muscular fatigue, loss of concentration, and high blood pressure. That's one reason why many health experts recommend a daily pill containing the water-solubles.

Minerals: Eat Your Sulphur, Johnny!

Minerals needed by the body are the same ones taken from the ground and used to manufacture automobiles, pipe, and refrigerators. Superman is the Man of Steel, but the rest of us can brag that, at least in part, we're Men and Women of Chromium, with magnesium muscles and iron blood cells. The only reason we don't clank when we walk or turn green like the Statue of Liberty is because the body uses only tiny amounts of minerals. No prospector is going to strike it rich by melting us down.

The cycle supplying minerals to the body begins in the earth. Plants growing in rich soil absorb minerals into their roots, stems, leaves, and fruits. Then humans either eat the plants or eat animals that have eaten the plants. Thus, corn on the cob and artichoke hearts transport minerals from the soil to human tissue.

Minerals are as essential to the body as vitamins. They participate in enzyme and hormone production, they give structure to teeth and bones, and they regulate muscle contractions and the conversion of food into energy. All the body's systems and tissues need them in large or small doses, as shown in Table 1.

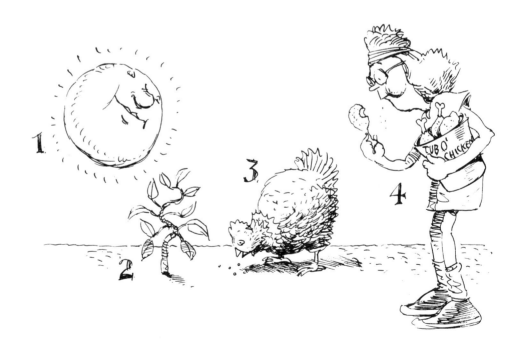

Table 1.

Essential Minerals

Needed in large amounts

Calcium	Potassium
Magnesium	Sodium chloride
Phophorus	Sulphur

Needed in trace amounts

Iron	Copper
Iodine	Fluoride
Cobalt	Manganese
Zinc	Molybdenum
Chromium	Selenium

The body needs all the minerals listed in Table 1 in varying amounts, which is another reason for a well-balanced diet. A lack of just one of the minerals can hurt the body. Insufficient calcium, for example, causes the bones to become brittle and may lead to foot trouble. If your diet is hit-or-miss, take a multiple mineral tablet for insurance.

The following minerals are of special importance to athletes:

SODIUM, POTASSIUM, CHLORIDE: THE ELECTROLYTES

If you've been around athletes for very long, you've heard the expression "electrolyte balance." Electrolytes are mineral compounds that maintain a balance of body fluids, which is vital to the athlete's cooling system.

Sodium (salt) is the largest mineral constituent of the blood. A low salt level can lead to dehydration because the body needs salt to retain water. This is why generations of coaches have passed out salt tablets to their troops. But they don't have to do that, because the body's need for salt can be easily met with a normal diet. In fact, the average American's salt intake is fifty times greater than it need be! It's rare to find an American who isn't salty enough.

While too little salt causes dehydration, too much can lead to dehydration, too. How? Excess salt increases urination to rid the body of the excess. This increased urination drains fluid from the body, and the lack of fluid can overload the cooling system and lead to heat stroke (see "The Cooling System").

Potassium departs the body through sweat and urination. Every time the body becomes dehydrated, it loses potassium, which is vital to cellular function in the following way: During exercise, heat must be eliminated from the working muscles. Like all the body's internal heat, it is eliminated through the bloodstream. Potassium acts to widen the blood vessels so that the increased blood supply eliminates the heat quicker. The immediate heat problem is solved, but the potassium problem won't be solved until more is digested.

A low level of potassium gives you that tired, run-down feeling you hear about in TV commercials. One of the more universally recommended mineral supplements is a potassium tablet.

Potassium also abounds in fruits and vegetables. Again, one of the best ways to quench your thirst after training or competition is with orange juice. You're resupplying the body with water and minerals lost through dehydration.

Chloride is as essential as sodium and potassium in maintaining electrolyte balance, but, because it's less easily lost through dehydration, it is less likely to be responsible for a deficient state in the body. Like sodium, chloride comes to us in sufficient quantities through a normal diet.

IRON

The red blood cells contain most of the body's iron, which is the primary ingredient of hemoglobin, the oxygen carrier. Iron deficiency results in not enough oxygen reaching the cells, which in turn means fatigue, listlessness, and inability to sustain aerobic exercise. Medically, this condition is called anemia; doctors check for it by taking a blood sample and counting the percentage of red blood cells. Anemia occasionally afflicts athletes but is easily corrected by ingesting plenty of red meat, spinach, and/or Geritol.

A MINERAL DIET

Fruits, vegetables, whole grains, and milk provide the best supply of essential minerals. But, like vitamins, they are not found in adequate amounts in any single food. And even with a diet that appears well-balanced, you may still be getting an inadequate supply. One reason: plants grown in soil that is mineral-deficient will produce fruits and vegetables that are equally deficient.

Taking a mineral tablet gives some insurance if the mineral tablet is properly put together, but that's a big "if." Some minerals must be in precise combinations to be absorbed by the body; some must be bound to other nutrients. And some, if taken alone, can cause physical problems such as ulcers or diarrhea. Unfortunately, some tablet manufacturers don't concern themselves with these problems. It's best that you ask a pharmacist to help you select the best brand.

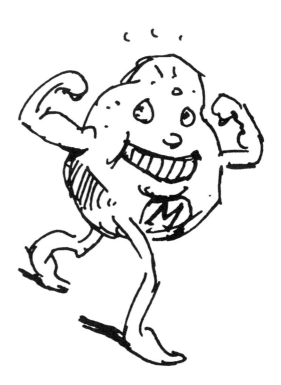

Athletes' Special Diets

High-Protein Diets: Spare the Spareribs

A few decades ago, there was near-unanimous agreement among athletic coaches about the wonders of protein. "Eat as much meat and eggs as your parents will tolerate, and then wash it down with a high-protein drink," was the familiar refrain. A generation has passed, and many coaches still say basically the same thing. Well, the fact is that any coach who tells you to eat T-bone steaks until they're coming out of your ears is wrong.

Unlimited omelettes and stacks of mutton chops are good for no one. The average person requires approximately sixty grams of protein a day—which might come from two eggs at breakfast, a fish

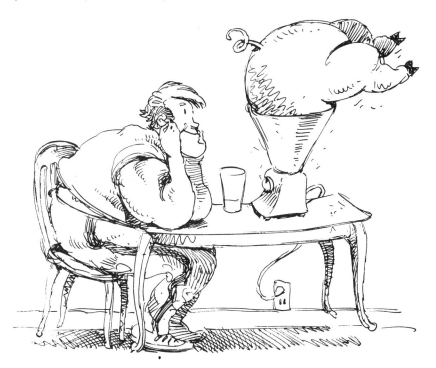

stick at lunch, and a lambchop at dinner. Larger amounts of protein could create problems.

"Protein is not stored by the body," says Dr. Ken Carter, a leading clinical pathologist. "When large amounts are ingested, tremendous strain is placed on the body's elimination system to rid itself of the excess."

But athletes regularly exert themselves more than the average person, so surely their recommended protein intake should be more than sixty grams a day, right? Wrong. Dr. Carter (whose views are widely shared in medicine) states: "Massive amounts of protein do nothing to help an athlete's performance or muscle growth. In fact, too much protein can actually harm an athlete. The athlete's delicate fluid and mineral balance can be affected by the elimination of the excess protein. The athlete suffers from protein poisoning."

Many athletes have consumed an average of *five hundred* grams of protein each day, but they've shown no visible improvement in performance while taking this health-hazardous route. The best bet is to stick to the recommended sixty-gram protein limit.

One final note: Since protein is not stored by the body, it is essential that you include it in your daily diet so it's on hand when needed to build and maintain muscle tissue. But in the case of protein, more is *not* best.

The No-Carbohydrate Diet Destroys Muscles

It seems that new diets are pushed at us every time we turn a page or flip a dial. The Scarsdale Diet, the Pritikin Diet, the Atkins Diet, the Martini Drinker's Diet. This painless way to lose weight, that way to shed ugly fat. Some have merit and some don't. Some not only don't work, but are dangerous as well. Particularly harmful to the athlete is the no-carbohydrate diet.

Bodybuilders were among the first athletes to experiment with this scheme, reasoning that completely avoiding foods containing carbohydrates would help eliminate fat while still allowing muscle growth. However, the diet is damaging because it causes not only the loss of fat but of muscle tissue as well.

"Studies have shown that a twelve-pound weight loss on a zero-carbohydrate diet will result in a four-pound loss in muscle tissue," says Dr. Homer Sprague, an expert in physical education and public health. "Losing the same twelve pounds on a low-carbohydrate diet (sixty grams a day) results in an insignificant loss in muscle tissue."

Why the difference?

"The body needs carbohydrates to metabolize protein," says Dr. Sprague, "and protein is the main ingredient of muscle fiber (not counting water), so without the carbohydrates, the muscle can't use the protein for building and maintenance."

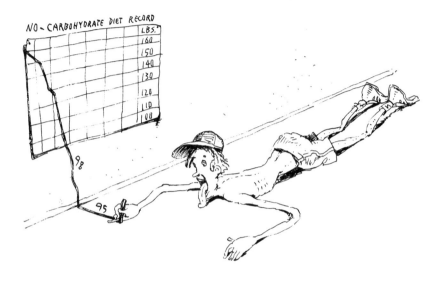

The Pre-Game Meal: Pasta Power

"There was a time," said the Los Angeles Rams' All-Pro defensive end Jack Youngblood, "when I would eat nineteen eggs and a big steak before a game. Now I'd sooner eat my helmet. I no longer believe in pre-game eating. All I have is three glasses of milk and ten cups of coffee."

"We don't believe in telling players what they have to eat," said Pittsburgh Steelers trainer Ralph Berlin, interviewed recently by sportswriter Melvin Durslag. "If a guy gets the notion in his head that he operates better on beef, we provide the beef. But, for the most part, our guys go for pancakes, biscuits, toast, eggs, ham, bacon, sausage, and baked potatoes."

The final feast—what, how much, and how long before the event? The athlete should make an intelligent choice that will benefit his performance, and the scientific consensus is that the choice should be high-carbohydrate foods, in moderate amounts, several hours before the tipoff, kickoff, faceoff, or whatever. In other words, make it lasagna instead of lambchops, spaghetti instead of steak.

Carbohydrates supply energy to the body more quickly than fats do. And they are more quickly digested and absorbed

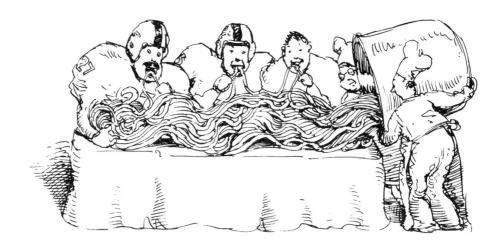

into the bloodstream. That's important, because digestion increases the supply of blood to the stomach, but during exercise muscles need more blood too. Therefore, it's best to have digested your mashed potatoes and gravy before the bell rings for the first round so that the muscles aren't competing with the stomach for the blood supply. You only have so much blood to spread around.

When should the pre-game meal be eaten? Too long before competition and you're hungry, too soon and digestive problems crop up. Assuming it's overwhelmingly carbohydrates—say, French toast with maple syrup—the meal should be put away three to four hours in advance. That's allowing time for the average rate of digestion. People differ, so personal experience is the final decider.

Should the meal be solid or liquid? Increasingly popular are canned liquid meals designed for weight-gain or weight-loss programs. They are nutritionally balanced and, more important for the competing athlete, more quickly digested than solid foods. A liquid meal is completely digested within two hours of consumption.

Not all carbohydrate foods are digested with the same ease. Many sports nutritionists believe that roughage foods like salads should be completely eliminated from the diet for two days prior to competition. That's because roughage foods put stress on the digestive system without adding their share of nutrients and energy. But don't avoid roughage all the time. It's needed by the body to keep the solid byproducts of digestion moving through the intestines.

Athletes are often gluttonous characters, washing down huge meals with equally huge amounts of liquid—which is a big mistake before competition. The larger the meal, the longer it takes to digest—with some unpleasant consequences (particularly including possible uncontrolled weight gain). Water, the basic ingredient of all liquids and most solid foods, can pass through the stomach and into the bloodstream at a rate of only about a quart each hour. The glutton who finishes off a gallon of milk during dinner has more than the milk's fats and proteins interfering with his digestion. That quantity of liquid won't leave his stomach for four hours.

In summary, the pre-game meal should be primarily carbohydrates, preferably liquid in moderate quantities. It should be consumed four hours before competition if it's solid food, two hours before if it's liquid. Forget the generations of hand-me-down advice that called for a steak dinner. Go modern.

Gaining Weight: Lift a Barbell, Not Your Fork

Gaining weight is easy in principle: simply put more calories down your throat than your body needs. But gaining the *right kind* of weight takes more effort than just raising a forkful of grits to your mouth. It takes hard training to add muscle instead of fat.

Any excess calories you swallow are stored as fat, whether they pass between your lips as fat, carbohydrates, or proteins. But an athlete does not want extra fat because it will slow his or her movements. It doesn't add to any push, pull, twist, or turn needed for any sport. Imagine Martina Navratilova competing in a tennis tournament with a twenty-five-pound lead belt around her waist. Yet many athletes compete with just such a handicap without realizing it.

Fat adversely affects the cardiovascular system too. The heart and bloodstream have that much more tissue to supply with nutrients and oxygen. That extra heart action and blood supply could be much better used to feed working muscles.

A gain in *muscular* body weight—attained by weightlifting or other workout systems discussed earlier in this book—may be desirable, because added muscle means added strength and faster movements. But be sure to gain muscular weight only in those muscles that affect your sport. A twenty-inch neck isn't going to help a bowler get more strikes. And Mr. Universe-sized biceps won't help a soccer player kick more goals.

Losing Weight: the Ali Way or the Sensible Way

In the fall of 1980, heavyweight boxing champion Larry Holmes defended his title against aging ex-champ Muhammad Ali in Las Vegas. Holmes had little trouble, and Ali's trainer, Angelo Dundee, threw in the towel before the start of the eleventh round.

Apart from age, Ali was fighting with another disadvantage. A few months before the fight he had weighed 256 pounds. By the official weigh-in he had gone down to 217½.

"[Ali] lost at least thirty-seven pounds in a very short period," said Keith Kleven, Holmes' physical therapist. "He went too far. When you lose so much so fast, after such a dramatic change in diet and physical activity, there is a drastic change in the function of the body's enzymes. Instead of losing fat, you begin to deplete muscle substance."

At a press conference later, Ali admitted he had taken

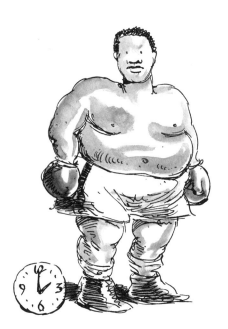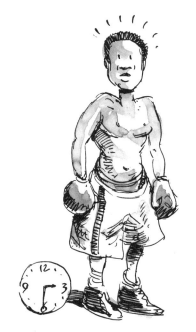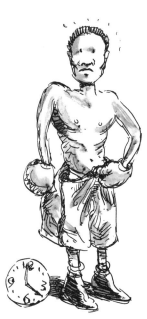

large doses of a drug named Thyrolar, usually prescribed for people with thyroid-gland deficiencies. Doctors said overdoses of the drug can cause dehydration and fatigue.

The lesson is clear: Don't try to lose fat too quickly or it will send shock waves throughout your body. Shock? Yes. The inside of your body is like the outside—used to doing the regular old things. One ingrained habit is the eating pattern you've developed over the years. Your body knows how to handle the customary amounts of food. When you suddenly change your habits, as by missing meals, your insides respond with headaches and hunger pangs. You feel tired because the digestive system and absorption process don't mesh gears. It takes time for the body to adjust its assembly line to the decreased flow of food. So let your body adjust slowly, and the fat will burn away with no bad side effects.

Most athletes want to be streamlined because any excess baggage slows and tires the body. Official racetrack handicappers have long used this fact to even their fields, adding weight to the Bold Rulers and Citations to slow them down. Pokey nags are assigned less weight.

Excess baggage is any body tissue that doesn't help the athlete's performance—usually fat, but sometimes muscle.

Fat is universally accepted as a problem. Unlike muscle, fat doesn't hold its own weight by helping to push and pull the body. It just hangs on for the ride.

Eliminating body fat, as we've seen, is easy in principle: just eat less than your body needs. Of course, the amount of food required varies from body to body and sport to sport. For example, a sumo wrestler uses more food than a jockey just to carry on the minimal body functions like sleeping and breathing. One sport might require the equivalent of two hundred calories of food each day, and another might require three thousand.

Precisely measuring the calories from food is difficult. So it's best to use a more general approach when beginning a weight-loss diet. Start by cutting out high-calorie foods (Cokes, cakes, pies). Eat smaller portions than are normal for you, and try eating more slowly. The scale will tell you if you've cut enough calories.

When trying to lose weight, don't neglect any of the essential nutrients. Depriving the body of one essential nutrient, remember, can affect the timing and efficiency of hundreds of chemical reactions.

Also excessive baggage are large muscles not involved in your sport. But how can you selectively lose tissue from an overly large muscle without also losing it from others? Easy. Muscles shrink, or atrophy, from disuse. The bigger the muscle, the quicker it weakens and shrinks from lack of use. And shrunken muscles weigh less. So if you don't continue to train already bulky muscles that aren't needed for your sport—if you're a soccer player and neglect your biceps, for example —the total effect will be to make you lighter.

Above all, be patient so that your body as a whole can cope with the changes.

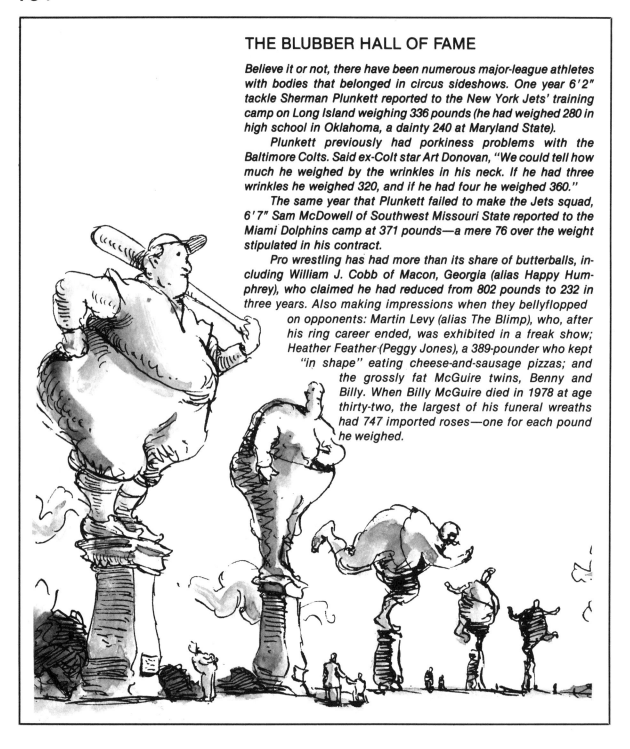

THE BLUBBER HALL OF FAME

Believe it or not, there have been numerous major-league athletes with bodies that belonged in circus sideshows. One year 6'2" tackle Sherman Plunkett reported to the New York Jets' training camp on Long Island weighing 336 pounds (he had weighed 280 in high school in Oklahoma, a dainty 240 at Maryland State).

Plunkett previously had porkiness problems with the Baltimore Colts. Said ex-Colt star Art Donovan, "We could tell how much he weighed by the wrinkles in his neck. If he had three wrinkles he weighed 320, and if he had four he weighed 360."

The same year that Plunkett failed to make the Jets squad, 6'7" Sam McDowell of Southwest Missouri State reported to the Miami Dolphins camp at 371 pounds—a mere 76 over the weight stipulated in his contract.

Pro wrestling has had more than its share of butterballs, including William J. Cobb of Macon, Georgia (alias Happy Humphrey), who claimed he had reduced from 802 pounds to 232 in three years. Also making impressions when they bellyflopped on opponents: Martin Levy (alias The Blimp), who, after his ring career ended, was exhibited in a freak show; Heather Feather (Peggy Jones), a 389-pounder who kept "in shape" eating cheese-and-sausage pizzas; and the grossly fat McGuire twins, Benny and Billy. When Billy McGuire died in 1978 at age thirty-two, the largest of his funeral wreaths had 747 imported roses—one for each pound he weighed.

RENOWNED GLUTTONS

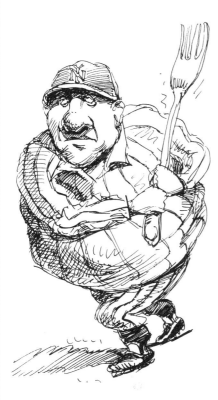

Babe Ruth, famous for hitting home runs, was just as good at handling a knife and fork as he was at swinging a bat. "He awed people with the amount of food he could eat," said Ping Bodie, a baseball contemporary. "Anybody who eats three pounds of steak and a bottle of chili sauce for a starter has got me."

Accounts of Ruth's eating feats were often exaggerated, but Robert Creamer, in his fine biography, Babe, The Legend Comes to Life, *verified that Ruth's appetite was indeed enormous: "A report of one dinner says he had an entire capon, potatoes, spinach, corn, peas, beans, bread, butter, pie, ice cream, and three or four cups of coffee. He was known to have eaten a huge omelet made of eighteen eggs and three big slices of ham, plus half a dozen slices of buttered toast and several cups of coffee."*

Here's a recent pregame meal devoured by Oakland Raiders defensive end John Matuszak (six-foot-eight and more than 270 pounds), as reported in the Los Angeles Times: *"ten eggs, seven slices of bacon, a chunk of ham, eight slices of toast, and a fourteen-ounce steak."*

Another football lineman, Ernie Ladd, who played in the National Football League at close to three hundred pounds (he's now a wrestler), won the first Golden West Eating Contest in 1963. Among the spectators were some of his teammates, who held up a placard that said, "Eat his arm off, Big Ern." Ladd's prizes: a heifer calf, which he probably ate that night for a bedtime snack, and a red-velvet championship belt, which probably wasn't big enough to fit around him.

You Can't Jiggle the Suet Away

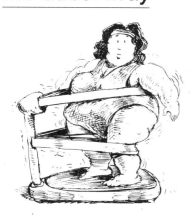

It would be dandy if Benny the Blimp could simply step into or strap himself into some vibrating machine and daydream while his huge waistline was shaken down to a svelte size. But that's impossible. Sauna wraps, massage, rubber clothing, or vibrating belts won't sweat, rub, shake, wiggle, jiggle, or tickle the fat away. Spot-reducing gadgets absolutely do not work.

Diet is the only way to get rid of extra fat. And diet removes fat uniformly from all parts of the body.

Fat cells are food-energy deposits placed throughout your innards. When the body needs more get-up-and-go than has been taken in as food, the bloodstream busily gathers fat from *all over the body* to supply energy to any muscle, bone, or nerve that's in need. The energy is not taken from any one deposit.

Broccoli Versus Beefsteak

Strict vegetarians—people who not only don't eat meat, but don't consume milk or eggs either—are rare. They live on fruits, vegetables, grains, nuts, and seeds. The danger with this practice is deficiency of vitamin B-12, which can be obtained only in tiny quantities from wheat germ, soybean powder, sprouts, and rare seaweeds. A prolonged lack of B-12 leads to general fatigue, anemia, and muscle weakness—symptoms that even a croquet player is better without. Small amounts of milk products, or B-12 tablets, are all that is needed to supply the body with an adequate supply of that vitamin.

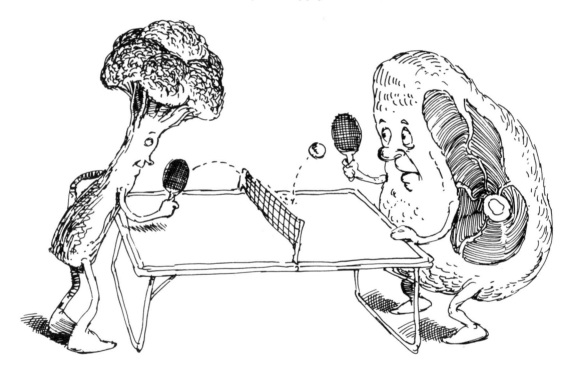

More common are "lacto-" or "ovo-lacto" vegetarians, who eat egg and dairy products, and people who merely avoid "red meat" but do eat fish and fowl.

Vegetarians argue that they have better general health than meat eaters, which may be true. It is certainly true that vegetarians have about half the meat eaters' level of saturated fats in their blood and thus have less chance of suffering from heart disease and high blood pressure.

But—Popeye and his spinach fixes to the contrary—there is no evidence that vegetarianism will make an athlete put the shot farther or bowl more strikes.

Beverages

Should Caffeine Be Outlawed?

Lots of people have to have their morning cups of coffee to face the day. Coffee jolts them awake. For the same effect, more and more athletes are drinking coffee during training and competition. Why? Because the beverage contains a natural stimulant, caffeine, which quickens reflexes, increases muscle strength and endurance, and speeds up the communication between the brain and the muscles.

However, this is not a sales pitch for Maxwell House or Yuban. Too much caffeine will excite the nervous sytem to the point of making the athlete ultranervous. And when the stimulation wears off, a mild physical and mental depression sets in.

An immediate problem with caffeine is that it increases urine production, acting as a diuretic that can slightly dehydrate the body. And if the caffeine comes in the form of hot coffee or hot tea, it can add to the body's heat-control problems, particularly on a hot day. Like any other internal body heat, this extra heat must be eliminated through evaporation, which leads to more dehydration.

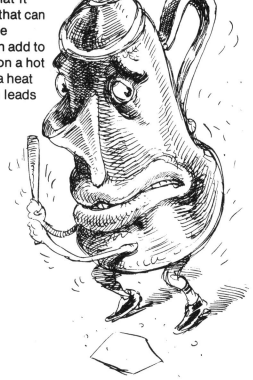

Something else to consider is caffeine's legality. Some sports organizations have outlawed it as a stimulant, along with amphetamines—and for the same basic reason: a stimulant not indigenous to the human body gives any athlete who uses it an unfair advantage in competition.

Not-So-Soft Drinks

Coffee and tea are not the only drinks that contain caffeine. Most of the so-called soft drinks have it, too. Our word cola comes from the name of an evergreen tree, cola or kola, that grows in Africa, India, and the West Indies. The nuts or seeds from the cola tree contain twice as much caffeine as coffee beans! However, since so many other things are mixed up in soft drinks, a Coca-Cola or Pepsi-Cola doesn't have as strong a stimulating effect as a cup of coffee.

The "Coca-" part of the "pause that refreshes" wasn't put in the name just because it sounded good. Coke's syrup used to be made not only from cola nuts but also from the dried leaves of the South American coca plant, the source of cocaine. Elderly people who worked at drug-store soda fountains years ago remember when cola was a combination of a brown syrup base from a jar and carbonated water from a spigot. They also remember a few regular customers who came in several times a day to eat the syrup with a spoon. Coca-Cola long ago changed its recipe, which is still a closely guarded secret.

Soft drinks also contain sweeteners, either sugar (up to five teaspoons in every eight-ounce can or bottle) or saccharin. Now, the body *needs* some form of sugar—it is the only thing the brain and nervous system burn for energy—but many Americans overdo consumption of processed sugar to a ridiculous extent. One recent study showed that the average person in the U.S.A. consumes more than one hundred and fifty grams of sugar a day.

Scientists have linked this colossal sweet tooth, "our most common addiction," to tooth decay, kidney disease, heart disease, high blood pressure, ulcers, diseases of the colon, diabetes, and behavior disorders.

Hence, the high sales figures for diet or sugar-free soft drinks such as Tab, Diet Pepsi, Pepsi Light, Diet-Rite Cola, etc., are not surprising. These drinks use saccharin, which is about five hundred times sweeter than sugar. It is not used by the body, so it doesn't add weight. But the U.S. government is not fond of it. Diet drinks using it have to carry this warning: "Use of this product may be hazardous to your health. This product contains saccharin, which has been determined to cause cancer in laboratory animals."

Save Alcohol for the Rubdown Table

Bourbon, tequila, beer, Scotch, gin, rum—they're all right in moderation. But alcohol is a poor source of energy. It's loaded with calories, yes, but they are "empty" calories, because they cannot be used as a direct source of energy. Alcohol must be converted to glucose before it can supply any vim, and that conversion is slow (about one ounce per hour). Yet it also takes a long time for the body to eliminate the alcohol from the bloodstream, and that which remains has a highly detrimental effect. The notion of exercising to hasten the metabolism of alcohol—a popular theory in some circles—is wrong and may be dangerous. Opportunities for injury to a person engaging in athletic activity while "under the influence" are so numerous as to imply strong self-destructive impulses in anyone who tries it.

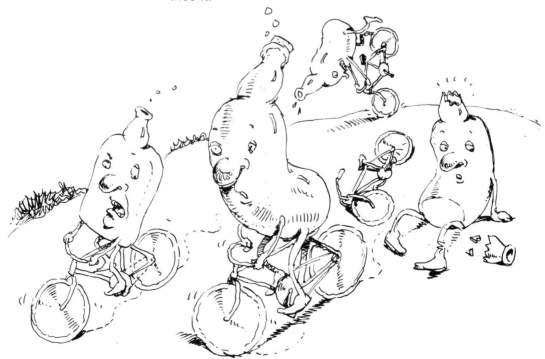

While a highball acts like a stimulant at first, it is actually a depressant to the central nervous system, inhibiting the blood's ability to transport oxygen to the cells and thus hindering athletic performance. Simply put, it dulls the senses.

Alcohol also has a dehydrating effect, widening the blood vessels in the skin and increasing heat loss. And it can be acutely addictive. A major-league pitcher and a major-league catcher both admitted in 1980 that they were alcoholics. The famous wrestling villain, Gorgeous George, wouldn't or couldn't give up booze and literally drank himself to death.

Most athletes know the bad effects of alcohol and use it only socially and occasionally. A survey of runners competing in the 1977 New York marathon showed that regular alcohol consumers were in a minority of 22 percent, while 59 percent were only occasional drinkers and 19 percent were teetotalers.

Cade's Gatorade

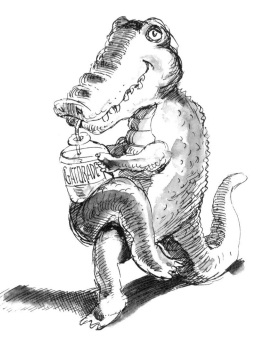

Gatorade is marketed by Stokely-Van Camp, Inc., of Indianapolis, but it was invented by a University of Florida professor of medicine, Dr. Robert Cade, who first called it Cade's Ade and Cadé's Cola. Stokely-Van Camp (famous for its canned pork and beans) does not squeeze alligators to get the liquid; the product's name comes from the university's sports teams, the Gators. Stokely-Van Camp considered calling it Thirst-Aide, Quench, and Super-Star before electing to keep the name chosen by Cade.

Gatorade and its imitators can be found in virtually every supermarket in the country now, but it was semi-revolutionary stuff when first used by athletes in a game in 1965 (Florida versus Louisiana State in football). Back then it was a clear liquid and tasted as if it had just been dipped out of Tampa Bay. Today it's sweeter, comes in lemon-lime and orange flavors, and has colors that reach out and grab shoppers.

Gatorade's ingredients sound to the layman's ear like something from a mad scientist's beaker of poison: glucose, sodium phosphate, citric acid, sodium citrate, and potassium citrate—all ingredients of electrolytes—to improve electrolyte balance. But don't let the fine print on the label scare you. Says Cade: "Gatorade is a beverage which quenches thirst, replaces the vital substances lost in perspiration—water, sodium, potassium—and is absorbed considerably faster than water."

Gatorade and similar products are good over ice and help prevent dehydration. (See an earlier essay, "The Disadvantage of Not Being a Camel.")

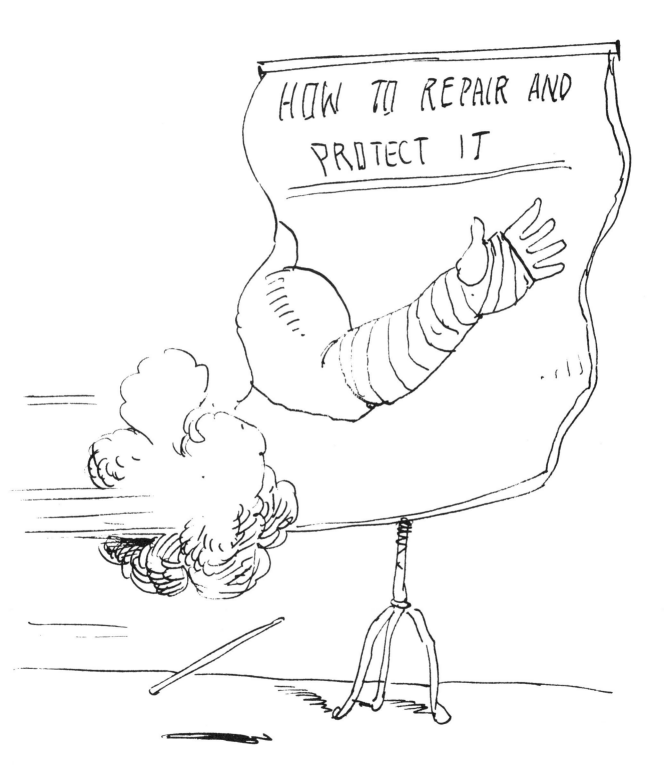

Introduction:
No Injury Is Routine

Athletes place extraordinary demands on their bodies—think of the midair acrobatics of basketball player Paul Westphal of the Seattle SuperSonics or the battering-ram runs of any National Football League fullback. The results are often injuries to themselves or others. Tennis players frequently get sore elbows. Basketball players, leaping dozens of times in a quarter, often twist their ankles when they land on other people's feet. But although strains, sprains, and bruises become *common,* they should not be treated as *routine*. Athletes can easily fall into the trap of treating injuries carelessly.

A minor injury can cause major problems if untreated or poorly treated. Every injury should be considered something of an emergency, calling for immediate, correct treatment.

Many of the short essays in this section include generally accepted methods of emergency treatment. Whether self-administered or performed by a trainer, coach, or doctor, the procedures are applicable to the usual athletic injuries. They should be used during the first forty-eight hours after the athlete is hurt.

But first the most important rule. Whenever the athlete is hurt, he or she should stop the activity. One more shot, jump, or swing can lead to a more serious injury. A small tear can stretch to a bigger tear, or worse.

If the injury is accompanied by muscle bleeding, continuing the movements will maintain or increase the already high level of blood circulation to the injured muscle tissue. This seeping blood causes swelling, which limits flexibility in the injured area. The seepage is also responsible for those nasty-looking black-and-blue marks that follow the swelling.

(Keep in mind, too, that injuries don't just occur in the big-time sports. Take the widespread incidence of Frisbee finger, for instance. Dr. Stancil E. D. Johnson discusses it at length in his *Frisbee, A Practitioner's Manual and Definitive Treatise*. ("It constitutes damage to the fingernail and associated structures as a result of the impact of a Frisbee on the tip of a finger," writes Dr. Johnson, who goes on to describe the worst type, or Grade III Frisbee finger, which is complete separation of the nail from the underlying bed.)

There are some healthy doses of preventive medicine prescribed here, too: how to protect the body in athletics as much as possible and—probably the most vital service we can perform in this book—some substances to avoid. Too many athletes think a pill, needle, beverage, or weed is some sort of magical shortcut to a goal, when in fact it may be a shortcut to permanent damage or death.

General Injury Treatment and Rehabilitation

The Iceman Cureth . . . and Other Trainers' Lore

Trainers probably use more ice than bartenders. That's because applying an icebag or other cold compress to an injured area of the body reduces swelling in all kinds of injuries. The application of cold constricts, or narrows, the broken blood vessels. That means less bleeding into the healthy tissue, and less bleeding leads to less swelling and less pain.

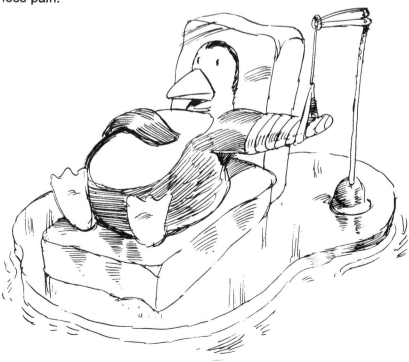

Throughout the two-day period following a muscle injury, cold should be applied in cycles of thirty minutes on and thirty minutes off. You're probably not going to have the stamina or patience to do it around the clock—or the discomfort tolerance to endure applications lasting longer than thirty minutes—but do try to do as many thirty-minute cycles as you can. The more frequently you apply the cold, the shorter and less severe the bleeding.

It's best to use a commercial icebag or ice cubes wrapped in a towel. The surface of the bag or towel acts as a safety buffer. Don't apply freezing ice directly to your warm skin. You don't need frostbite added to your troubles.

Along with giving the injured area enough ice to make it feel like a penguin wing, wrap it with an elastic bandage. Again, the reason is to reduce swelling from the broken blood vessels in the injured muscle tissue. The compression from the bandage won't permit blood to seep into surrounding tissue.

The wrap should be applied tightly enough to act as a dam against the swelling, but not tightly enough to block normal circulation. If a bone break is suspected, the wrap should be replaced by a splint if possible until professional medical help arrives.

Raising the injured part above the level of the heart will slow down loss of blood from the damaged vessels. Of course, not all injuries are located such that this piece of advice can be followed. But when possible, elevate the injury while applying cold and a compression wrap. Every little bit helps to stop the damaging swelling.

Pain's Message

Dave Cowens, the outstanding basketball center from Florida State University, retired from the Boston Celtics in 1980 after slightly more than ten full pro seasons. He had been hampered by foot ailments. Cowens wrote his own career obituary, which ran in both Boston newspapers, and one sentence stood out: "I do not believe in taking medication which many others utilize to mask the pain and allow them to play more years and earn more income."

Contrast Cowens with another fine center, the exuberant Bill Walton of UCLA, the Portland Trail Blazers, and the San Diego Clippers. Walton never played a full season from the time he turned pro in 1974 to the unhappy day in 1981 when his doctor said his playing career was over. Again, the main problem was foot ailments (although he also had knee surgery and broken wrists).

Walton's left foot was hurting midway through the 1978 season, when he was still with the Trail Blazers. It turned out to be a stress fracture, and he missed the entire 1978–79 season. His attorneys subsequently filed a $5.6-million lawsuit against a Trail Blazers doctor, a clinic, and twenty unnamed persons, claiming that the doctor and the clinic "carelessly and negligently examined, diagnosed, treated, tested, and cared for the plaintiff. . . ."

The suit, which is still pending, claims the doctor and clinic negligently prescribed oral doses of pain-killing and anti-inflammatory drugs and negligently injected Walton with a pain-killing drug.

The San Diego Clippers signed him for the 1979–80 season, but protected themselves by taking out an insurance policy on him with two British companies, Lloyd's of London and Home Insurance. Walton played only fourteen games that season and none at all in 1980–81. The Clippers sought to collect on their policy, were turned down, and filed a $12.5-million suit against the insurers.

Green Bay Packers placekicker Chester Marcol has charged that the pro football club gave him Novocaine, a pain killer, for a groin injury and had him kick against the New York Jets in a 1979 game. He said kicking with the injury resulted in the muscle tearing. Packers Coach Bart Starr and trainer Domenec Gentile denied that any medical risk had been taken with Marcol.

How quickly a sidelined athlete resumes training depends on the extent of his or her injury. There is no average time. It varies from person to person and injury to injury. The individual—whether athlete, doctor, or trainer—will have to be the judge. And one of the most significant indicators on which to base the judgment is pain.

Pain is nature's warning system. If walking on a sprained ankle causes pain a day or month after the injury, it's too early to resume all-out workouts. If pain is absent, you should resume training with caution, gradually placing increased demands on the ankle. An all-out effort, even without the painful warning, can lead to sudden collapse of an injured, unprepared muscle. Be sure not to overload a muscle after an injury.

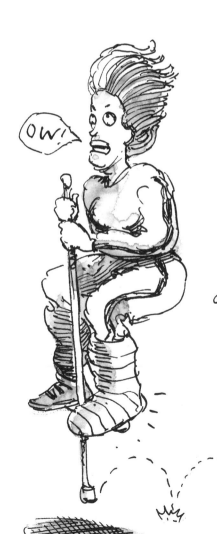

R & R for Recovering Muscles

Earvin (Magic) Johnson, the Los Angeles Lakers basketball star, injured a knee early in the 1980-81 season and didn't get back in action until mid-February. He probably could have returned earlier, but he wisely took his time and made sure the muscles in the injured leg were at least on the way back to top shape.

An unused muscle quickly atrophies and loses strength. Even healthy muscles can't match top-level performance after a period of inactivity. The process doesn't take long; the downward spiral begins after several days of rest.

To compensate for this strength loss, many trainers recommend a weight-training program to restrengthen the muscles. The basic principle of a restrengthening program is the same as a program to build up muscles from scratch—progressive resistance. The primary difference is that emphasis is placed on the injured area.

Obviously, an injured leg that has been in a cast for several weeks doesn't have the same capacity as the leg that has been hopped about on. So the training program must be tailored to compensate for the lopsided strength capacity brought about by the injury. In weight training, this can be done by requiring the recently injured leg to push or pull less weight than the sound one. Since the strong leg is already operating at or close to its full capacity, the weak leg will improve more rapidly and—with increasing amounts of weight assigned to it at each workout—will gradually "catch up" to the uninjured leg.

Similar adjustments can be made in other kinds of training programs. Runners, for instance, can wear different weights strapped to their ankles during their workouts, thus adapting their daily workload to the changing needs of a leg being built back up from injury.

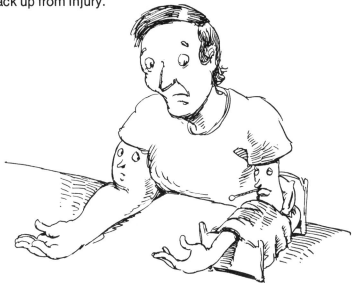

Healing Heat

Ice applied to an injury during the first two days is helpful, but after forty-eight hours the athlete should move from the Arctic to the tropics, so to speak. Most doctors and trainers recommend heating the injured area during the recuperative period—the theory being that heat will increase circulation, which in turn will deliver more of the blood's healing agents to the injury.

Heat is useful for virtually any type of athletic injury and can be delivered in many ways. The precise method is decided by the depth of the injury. A near-surface bruise—say, Houston Oilers running back Earl Campbell suffering from a sore thigh after a vicious tackle—can be treated with surface applications: perhaps hot towels, hydroculators (small, simple, portable devices that retain heat), heating pads, or heat lamps.

If a bruised, strained, or torn muscle happens to be deep within the limb or thorax (that part of the trunk between the neck and abdomen), the surface application of heat won't reach the injured tissue. That's because flesh is a poor conductor of heat. So it's necessary to use a more sophisticated device, an ultrasonic vibrator, which produces hundreds of thousands of sound vibrations per minute. These have an effect that is similar to heat. One of the drawbacks is that ultrasound equipment, primarily because of its excessive cost, isn't commonly available in training rooms. You usually have to visit a doctor's office to get zapped ultrasonically.

Another method of producing increased circulation—similar to that produced by heat—is massage, which can be used in place of ultrasound for most body areas.

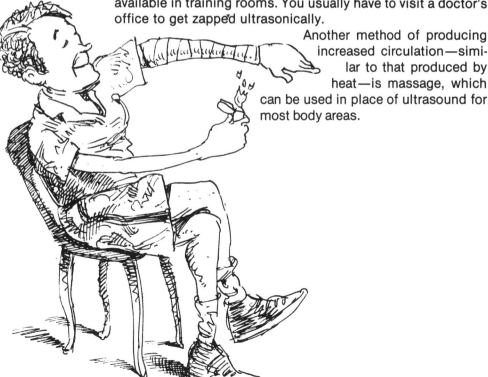

Don't Be Dizzy

In major-league baseball's 1937 All-Star Game, pitcher Jay Hanna (Dizzy) Dean, who had been the National League's most valuable player in 1934 and who had boasted a 24-13 record in '36, was hit in the foot by a line drive off the bat of Earl Averill. He suffered a broken toe.

Dean tried to come back to the St. Louis Cardinals too soon after the injury. He favored the toe, which caused him to alter his pitching motion and develop a sore arm. He was never a great pitcher again. His record was 13-10 in 1937, and he never won even as many as ten games in any one season again, although years later (in 1953) he was elected to the Baseball Hall of Fame.

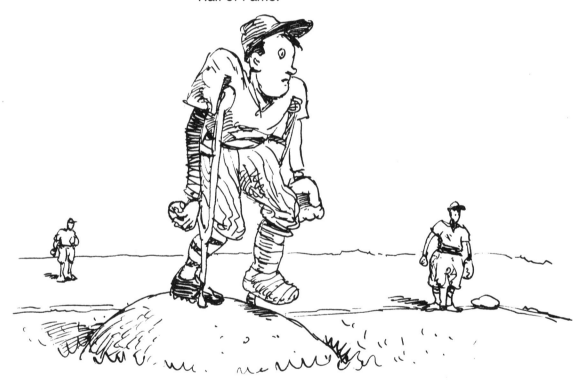

Too many athletes have lost or shortened their careers by being too anxious to get back into action. It's impossible to precisely determine the extent of any injury. Trainers, coaches, athletes, and doctors don't have the diagnostic tools or expertise to understand all the subtleties of a subsurface injury. It's preposterous to think otherwise.

The overriding concept in dealing with injuries is caution. It is the beginning and end of treatment.

Injury Prevention

Sleeping and Eating to Avoid Injuries

Diet and rest are two parts of the athlete's basic foundation that play an important role in preventing physical problems. Without the right eating and sleeping habits, muscles weakened by undernourishment may falter under stress or—worse—tear; reactions dulled by lack of sleep may fail in the clutch. Athletes who do use their knives and forks intelligently, and are careful about getting their rest, not only will improve their performances but will also lower their chances of getting hurt.

Not every injury can be avoided any more than every forest fire can be prevented, but these tips on off-the-field, out-of-the-pool preparation will help your chances to be injury-free. They require little, if any time, so why not try them?

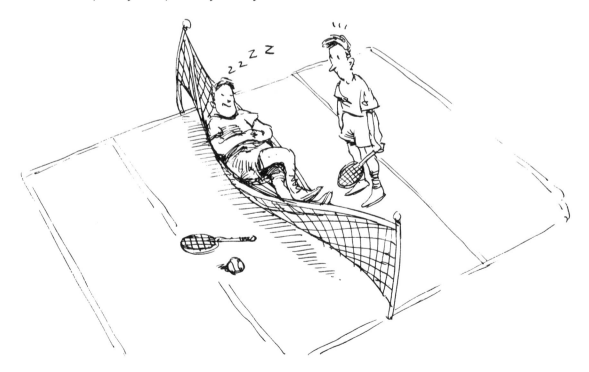

FOOD

The body manufactures thousands of different chemical compounds from the two dozen essential nutrients we get in the food we eat. Missing just one of these nutrients through improper food selection starts a chain reaction that limits production of hundreds of these needed compounds. For example, failure to eat foods containing potassium—a nutrient we lose every time we sweat—results in a shortage of compounds needed for the athlete's muscular efficiency. Making even customary demands on undernourished muscles can cause injury.

LIQUID

Dehydration and heat stroke are two of the more common physical problems associated with liquids in the athlete's diet. Of course, the athlete's performance is hurt long before a low water level becomes a medical problem.

The athlete's nerve-impulse accuracy and temperature are adversely affected when he's as little as two quarts low on water. And he can lose more than a *gallon* during an hour of training or competing. How does that cause injuries? An inaccurate impulse can lead to too much or too little muscle contraction during a crisis—say, Houston Oiler Earl Campbell bearing down on your linebacker position—and POP goes the muscle, tearing itself or a tendon and incapacitating one suffering athlete.

PRE-GAME MEAL

Know what and when to eat. That last meal before training or competing has an effect on the body's ability to handle physical stresses. Your blood should not be too busy with digestion to supply needed oxygen to the working muscles. (Under the stress of competition or training, tissue damage can result if the muscles are deprived of energy-providing oxygen.) And the digested food should be of the highest energy-producing groups of foodstuff—primarily carbohydrates, to be specific.

REST

Training and competition often involve maximum physical demands being placed on the body. Picture Tracy Caulkins straining to set a world record in the individual medley, or Evonne Goolagong Cawley serving at match point at the U.S. Tennis Open. Can their bodies perform to maximum capacity if tired? Of course not.

Frogs and salamanders don't need to sleep, but human beings do. For a long time scientists believed that sleep was the time when the body replaced worn-out cells and repaired damaged tissues. That has turned out not to be true—just as much repair work goes on during waking periods. The brain doesn't take any time off either; free from directing the body's walking, sitting, eating, etc., it dreams!

Most researchers break up sleep into four stages. Stage one is a sort of twilight zone in which the person has no directed thoughts. Stage two: the brain becomes more active and there is some dreaming. Stage three: the body is now totally relaxed; pulse and temperature are down. Stage four: the person is in *delta sleep*, the deepest phase (this is when a child's bed-wetting is most likely to occur). People don't just sink into stage four and stay there until awakening; they move up and down among the stages.

There is no prescribed amount of sleep everyone needs. Eight hours is not the magical amount. Each athlete has to figure out what is best for him or her. Too little sleep will cause irritability and erratic reaction time, opening the door to a multitude of misjudgments and missteps that would easily be avoided by a well-rested athlete whose timing was "on." And the American Cancer Society says the longest sleepers (ten hours or more) are more likely to have heart attacks and fatal strokes.

(All birds and mammals sleep, and it is interesting to note that man's twin in sleeping habits is the mole, which sleeps about eight hours out of every twenty-four and emits brain waves similar to ours.)

Rest doesn't mean just sleep, however. The muscles need rest from physical demands in order to recuperate for another round of demands. If inadequately rested muscles are forced to endure maximum demands, they frequently sustain injuries ranging from tears all the way to ruptures. You actually can overtrain.

Safety Equipment: More Fun than a Puck Sandwich

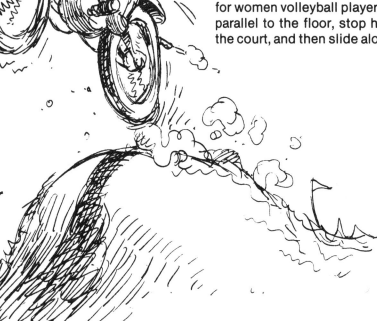

Some athletes avoid using safety equipment for reasons ranging from vanity to laziness. There was a time when goalies in the National Hockey League didn't wear masks. They thought it would be sissified and impair their vision, but eventually they got smart and decided puck sandwiches didn't taste good—especially when delivered at up to 120 miles an hour. (The masks are molded of fiberglass, with cutouts for eyes, nose, and mouth, and airholes on the sides.) Goalie Gerry Cheevers used to decorate his mask with drawings of stitches he *would* have received if he had played barefaced. The mask had more tracks on it than a railroad yard.

Then there is the occasional macho wrestler who actually *wants* the badge of his sport, a cauliflower ear, and refuses to wear any protective headgear. Eventually he'll receive a blow to the side of the head, causing a superficial hematoma (collection of blood) between the skin and the fibrocartilaginous skeleton of the ear. It will be red and sore as a boil at first, then stiff and unbendable and, yes, similar in appearance to a cauliflower except in color.

The sensible thing to do is take advantage of whatever safety equipment is available in your sport. Boxers use mouthpieces so they won't lose any teeth. Baseball catchers wear cups to protect their genitals, plus masks and chest protectors. Football players, bicycle racers, and motorcycle racers wear helmets. Mafia hit men wear bulletproof vests.

There are simple, common items of clothing that provide comfort as well as protection—e.g., athletic supporters for men and bras for women. Women boxers, for example, wear hard plastic bras. And there are specially padded bras available for women volleyball players, who—like the men—learn to dive parallel to the floor, stop hard-hit balls before their chests hit the court, and then slide along like playful seals.

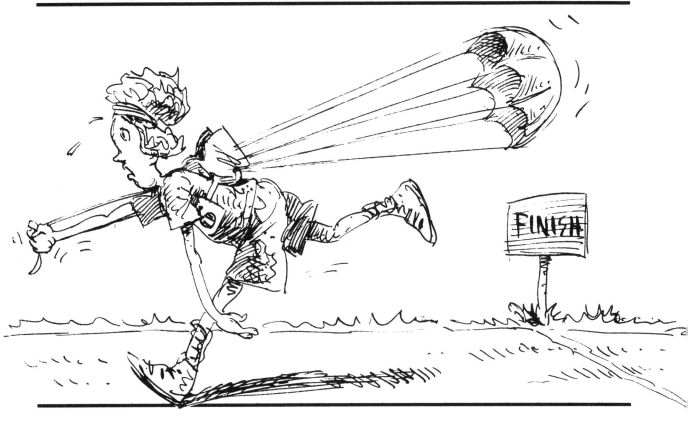

Cool Down!

Most athletes finish a game or workout and just plop or immediately undress and get in the shower. After the final buzzer, most professional basketball players walk to the locker room, sit on a stool or chair, and drink a cold beer or soda while they talk with each other or with sportswriters. A systematic approach to cooling down after exercise is neglected more often than not. Most athletes expect their bodies to return to normal without special help—and they might. But doing it that way could be costly.

Cooling down too quickly can lead to stiff muscles that are more prone to injury during the next workout. And it doesn't help the cardiovascular system to abruptly lower an elevated pulse rate.

If you have jogged three miles around the local high-school track, don't just walk back to your car and drive away when you're through. Walk a lap, then do some stretching exercises while your muscles are still warm and supple. James Fixx, author of *The Complete Book of Running*, says that when you stop, your pulse should be within twenty beats of what it is at rest.

Keep in Shape
All Year

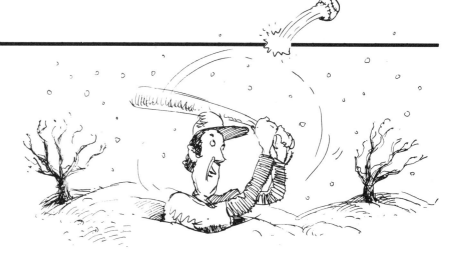

Apart from collisions—linebacker Jerry Robinson of the Phila-delphia Eagles getting blocked by Ron Yary of Minnesota, for instance—most athletic injuries come from placing too great a demand on an unprepared muscle. So it doesn't take a Rhodes scholar to figure out that athletes should report for their season in good shape. Obviously, a generally fit body has less trouble meeting start-of-season demands than an out-of-shape body.

Smart coaches have their players train in one way or another during the off-season, not only to work on weaknesses in technique but to improve strength—or at least prevent mus-cle atrophy, which is responsible for shortening many athletic careers.

Muscle atrophy (shrinking) results from placing less stress on the muscle than it's accustomed to handling. Muscle tissue is like the rest of the body's tissue (and the body as a whole) in that it works only as hard as it must.

Studies have indicated that strength can be maintained with as little as one isometric workout or two barbell workouts per week at about 90 percent of capacity. Endurance condition-ing follows a similar pattern; fewer workouts are needed to maintain high levels during the off-season. (The training essays in "How to Improve It" provide more detail on this topic.)

Warm Up and
Tune Up

Before Barbra Streisand goes on stage to perform, she warms up by doing some singing in her dressing room or somewhere backstage. At a concert, the cellists, piano players, and flutists tune their instruments right up to the moment the conductor taps his baton on the podium and signals the orchestra that it is time to begin.

The athlete should tune his *body* before performing (as described in a previous article, "Warm Up to Win"). This warm-up is just what the name implies—it actually raises the temperature of the muscles. Muscles that are warmed up a few degrees have greater strength and endurance capacity. This is true of animals as well as humans. At Santa Anita or Aqueduct, the thoroughbred horses are walked and galloped for several minutes before they enter the starting gate.

But warm-ups not only improve performance; they also help prevent injuries. Warming up routes a greater percentage of the oxygen-carrying blood to the working muscles, postponing fatigue. And it increases the amount of synovial fluid at the involved joints, which eliminates joint friction.

What types of warm-ups are best?

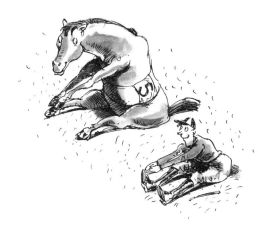

1. Stretching exercises to loosen your muscles.

2. Duplications of the motions of your sport or event—perhaps shooting at the basket or performing cartwheels. That way, you're sure to have warmed the muscles that actually will be used. It does no good to warm up leg muscles exclusively if you're going to be playing table tennis.

3. A number of repetitions—or duration of workout—that takes the weather into account. In warm weather (or in the gym), the muscles respond to a warm-up routine more quickly than in cold weather.

Remember: Whatever the slight difference in time required, a few minutes of warm-ups will cut down the potential for injury and misery.

Get a Grip on Yourself—with Tape

Treat old injuries with respect. A once-injured area is more likely to be hurt than a never-before-injured part of the body. Protecting the old injury might require nothing more than taping a chronically weak ankle (the ankle is the joint most susceptible to injury) or using a padded heel cup to protect a bruised heel. And there are more elaborate devices, including individually fitted braces.

Sportswriter Mike Littwin of the *Los Angeles Times* checked out the training staff of the USC football team and learned that it used a *mile* of tape a day, at a cost of about $35,000 a season! Taping an entire college football team the USC way takes two hours from first player to last, and it takes a trainer about a year to learn how to do it.

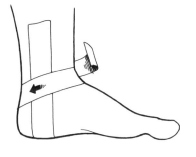

Most protective taping is done with plain ol' two-inch adhesive tape, laid over a thin layer of foam padding so that no tape actually touches the skin. There are many methods for applying the tape, each popular in a different area or a different field of athletics. For the ankle—which is the most commonly taped part of the body in most sports—the USC football trainers use the "Louisiana heel lock" taping system (don't ask!), which gives the most mobility without sacrificing protection. A typical method of ankle taping is illustrated in Figure 1.

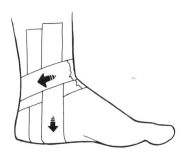
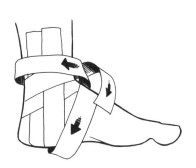
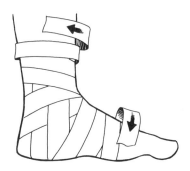

Fig. 1. *Protective taping prevents old injuries from acting up under stress.*

Dressing Right: Don't Wear a Parka in Panama

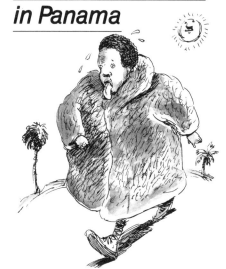

If your body is too hot or too cold, it doesn't perform to maximum efficiency. And if the body deviates more than a little from its normal internal temperature of about ninety-eight degrees (plus or minus two degrees), some very damaging things can happen.

Too warm an internal temperature speeds evaporation and can lead to dehydration, heat stroke, or breakdown of the body's protein structures.

Too low an internal temperature leads to constricted blood vessels and, in turn, greater potential for muscle and bone joint damage. (All the excess blood leaves the muscles to heat the core of the body.)

Clothing can help keep the body warm or cool, so choose the right garb for the weather and the sport. A marathon in a country near the equator should not be run in a fur coat. A bikini would not be appropriate for a sled-dog race in the Yukon. (Refer to the earlier essays in the section on the cooling system.)

Muscle Injuries

Myositis:
Stiff and Sore
the Next Morning

Dagwood Bumstead doesn't exercise much. Maybe he runs to catch the bus in the morning and walks to the office water-cooler several times a day. Then he decides to take part in the touch football game at the annual office picnic. He will be pleasantly tired afterward as he tears into the fried chicken and potato salad. But it won't be so pleasant the next morning when he tries to get out of bed. He'll be suffering from myositis.

Myositis is not a dread disease spread by bacteria from rotting toadstools. It is merely the fancy name for muscle soreness—that common pain most people wake up with the day after being a once-a-year left halfback. It is a general tenderness of major muscle groups, not the specific location pain that stems from a muscle tear or rupture.

If Bumstead could examine the tender areas with a subsurface microscope, he would find that the muscles were inflamed and mildly

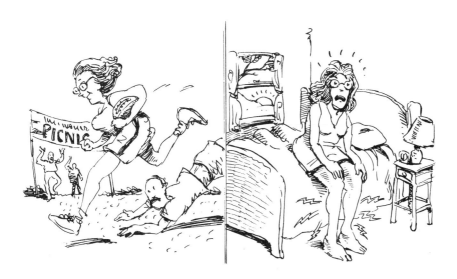

swollen. And he might find that some of the tissue had microscopic tears. If his individual muscle cells had lungs and vocal chords, he'd hear a chorus of pain with each movement.

Unlike strains and ruptures, the effects of myositis disappear more quickly if exercise is continued. It is painful to train with sore muscles, but the pain will depart with exercise—apparently because the increased circulation helps induce healing.

Cramping Your Style

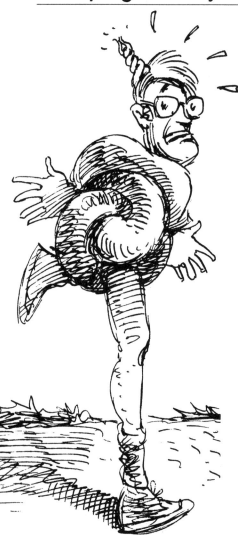

Two-man beach volleyball tournaments are grueling affairs, usually going on all day Saturday and all day Sunday. The sun beats down, and time and time again the athletes fling themselves around the rope-bordered court and churn through the sand to leap and spike. It is common at these events to see a player collapse on the sand in agony and frantically rub a muscle, usually in one leg.

The culprit is not a stinging beach insect, but a muscle cramp. A muscle cramp (or charleyhorse, or spasm) is a muscle contraction that lasts too long—a contraction that won't *un*-contract. In general it is the result of salt depletion, usually through sweating, but it can also result from muscle fatigue or injury.

Diagnosis is usually no problem because a cramp is easily recognizable as a painful, unexpected tightening of the muscle (quite often the calf at volleyball tourneys). The cramp may form a "lump," and it always hurts.

Since a cramp is a prolonged contraction, the prescribed treatment is to relax the muscle. That is most rapidly accomplished by stretching the muscle to its normal, relaxed position. For example, the arm bicep bends the elbow as it contracts. The proper treatment to relax the contracted bicep is to straighten the elbow in order to stretch the bicep. Similarly the volleyballer can relieve a calf cramp by pointing the toes toward the shin to stretch the offending muscle into submission.

After stretching, massaging the cramped muscle usually helps. Massage is simply a variation of relaxing the muscle through stretching. As the muscle is manipulated and stretched by the fingers, the muscle relaxes.

The muscle can be used immediately after the cramp subsides. However, caution is the best course if it returns, because that indicates it was caused by a slight muscle tear. And a slight muscle tear can become severe if the injured muscle is subjected to continued demands.

Strained Muscles: Torn and Painful

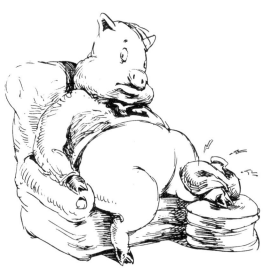

It is common in training rooms to hear talk—or moans—about a "pulled hamstring" or a "pulled groin muscle." A muscle pull is the same thing as a muscle *strain:* a partial tear across the width of the muscle fibers. The damaged muscle, like a similarly torn rubber band or rope, still works, but with less strength.

It's hard to distinguish a strained muscle from other muscle injuries described in this section. As in some of the other injuries, beneath the body's surface, at the point of the tear, the muscle is bleeding—resulting in surface swelling and lots of pain.

Even when the injury is correctly diagnosed, trainers and doctors may have difficulty figuring out how serious it is. The tear may be small or large, involving only a few fibers or the greater part of the muscle's width.

Treat a suspected muscle strain by applying an icebag to the injured area as soon after the injury as possible. The icebag helps control the internal bleeding and swelling that causes much of the pain. The ice treatment should be continued until the bleeding stops. When this happens, usually within forty-eight hours, reverse the treatment by applying heat. The heat acts to increase circulation to the injury, which is necessary to aid the body's natural healing processes.

Don't use the muscle for two days. Then, if you feel you can safely return to training, resume carefully. Easy does it.

Muscle Rupture: A Break No Athlete Needs

A muscle is called ruptured when it is completely severed (see Fig. 2). The general effect is like an extended rubber band, which, when cut, recoils in two different directions. Similarly, when a muscle is severed, it springs back and then hangs uselessly from the bones. It's painful just to *read* about. The victim suffers extreme pain and swelling, and the subsurface bleeding is greater than with a strain, because more tissue is torn.

Sometimes a ruptured muscle is misdiagnosed as a ruptured tendon, since both put a joint or limb out of commission. But most sports doctors can distinguish the difference by the location of the severest pain. If the injury is to a tendon, the pain will be closer to the tendon's insertion at the bone. If it's a ruptured muscle, the worst pain will be somewhere along its "belly" (i.e., the middle of the muscle, which is usually also its thickest part).

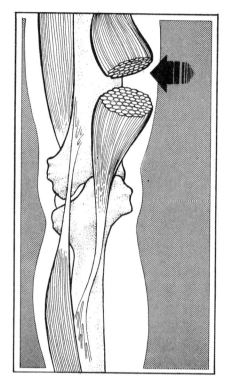

Fig. 2. *Sudden, gross overload of a muscle can cause a complete rupture.*

The athlete should quickly apply ice to the injured area. It won't mend anything, but it will hold down the swelling, and that, in turn, will help limit the pain.

Prompt medical treatment is essential for a ruptured muscle. The only possible cure is surgery to sew the severed ends together again. The longer the muscle is left damaged, the more atrophy will inhibit recovery, so prompt action is essential.

Near the end of the volleyball competition at the 1964 Olympics in Tokyo, Mike O'Hara of the American team was hurrying through his warm-up for a match. He leaped up at the net to spike and completely missed the ball, rupturing his right pectoral muscle (in the chest). Doctors later told him he had probably been pushing the muscle to the breaking point for years by constant spiking in beach and indoor tournaments.

O'Hara, now an official with the organizing committee for the '84 Games in Los Angeles, went for about a year without being able to spike in volleyball or serve in tennis before he finally underwent surgery to repair the injury.

All is not lost when an athlete ruptures a muscle. Surgery often leads to full recovery and renewed use, as it did in O'Hara's case.

Fortunately, a muscle rupture—which is usually caused by a sudden, gross overload—is much less common in sports than a muscle strain or partial tear—which is usually caused by a gradually increasing overstress. Weightlifters are among the few types of athletes who are likely to be subjected to conditions leading to complete muscle rupture.

If surgery is not considered appropriate for some reason, other things can be done to recondition the body for competition. If the muscle isn't vital to the athlete's sport, and if it's located so that it can be "isolated" from demands on it, the athlete's coach may recommend a slightly altered competitive technique to shift muscular demands to healthy muscles. Obviously, this is not possible in cases in which the ruptured muscle is essential to a particular event—say, a right-handed discus thrower's right bicep.

When the muscle has been surgically mended, the coach often refers the athlete to the trainer, who can devise a strength and flexibility program for the weakened area (the repaired muscle itself and others used in the same general movement). By strengthening the helping muscles, the athlete gives the recovering muscle an easier workload.

Hernia: An Intrusion that Hurts

A hernia—the protrusion, or bulging, of part of an intestine through a partial tear in the muscle wall of the abdomen—is sometimes called a rupture, but that is misleading because nothing is actually severed. Hernias are common among boy infants and old men, especially sedentary or bedridden old men with weak muscles. Exercise helps to prevent a hernia. Hard work or lifting heavy objects won't cause one unless there already is a weakness.

An *inguinal hernia* is a bulge into the scrotum (the sack holding the testicles) or the labia of the vagina. It is more common in boys ("Turn your head and cough," says the doctor as he probes). A *femoral hernia* is a bulge into the area where blood vessels go into the leg.

A hernia can be held in place by a truss (a tight binding) but can be cured only by surgery.

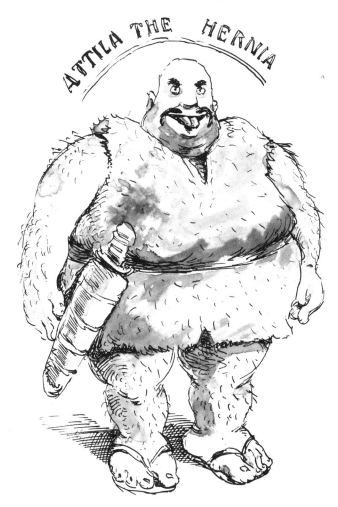

Scar Tissue: Mother Nature's Stitches

Scar tissue is the body's way of stitching together torn muscle. Unfortunately, this dense, fiber-filled connective tissue, when subjected to athletic stress, can cause a lot of pain and damage to surrounding muscle.

A persistent pain in an area near an old injury indicates that the lack of flexibility in scar tissue is the cause. How? Each time the athlete uses the muscle, the healthy muscle tissue must overstretch to compensate for the relatively rigid scar tissue. This overstretching of the healthy tissue causes the pain. And, if the stretching goes too far, the muscle is ripe for more tears or ruptures. It's a vicious circle—tears develop scar tissue which brings on more tears.

The goal in overcoming the scar-tissue handicap is to increase the muscle's overall flexibility without adding new injuries in the process. It's best to begin with mild stretching, then gradually do more intensive stretching in subsequent workouts. Start easy and progress; don't start fast and regress.

Scar tissue played a part in the problems of Pitcher Tommy John, a Los Angeles Dodgers star who later played for the New York Yankees. After his left elbow was repaired in 1974 (discussed earlier in "The Body's Connectors"), doctors discovered that scar tissue had cut off the ulnar nerve in his pitching arm and his hand had become crippled as a result. By the time surgeons unblocked the nerve, there had been quite a bit of atrophy.

But John never lost his determination and positive frame of mind. "Tommy did everything in the world," said a Dodger coach. "He rigged up a little harness to his hand to help him hold the ball. At night he stuck tongue depressors on his fingers to straighten them out.

"The amazing thing was he never had a doubt he was going to pitch again. I'm sure he had his moments, but he sure never let anyone know it. He went about his business like there was no doubt about it, like he was right on schedule."

Bone Injuries

Broken Bones: Hairline Fracture and Worse

Any of a human being's more than two hundred bones can be damaged if hit or twisted hard enough, and broken and bruised bones are common in sports. If there is any indication of a bone injury, professional diagnostic equipment (usually an X-ray machine) is needed. Don't try home treatment. Herbs, acupuncture, or incantations are fine for some things, but they aren't likely to help mend bone breaks.

In a *complete fracture* (see Fig. 3a), the bone is broken into separate pieces. the break leaves jagged edges that can pierce the surrounding tissue or even protrude through the skin.

A complete fracture requires emergency medical treatment. But until the doctor arrives, the injured area should be packed in icebags to keep swelling to a minimum. And don't place any stress

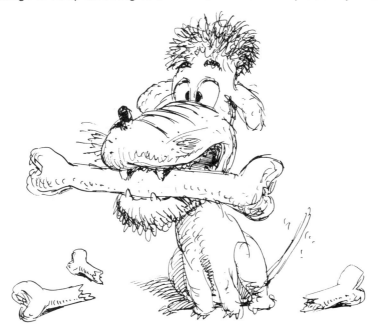

on the fracture (like walking on a broken leg), as this can cause the bone to push through more tissue—and possibly even cut a major nerve or artery.

A *stress fracture* is a slight crack in the surface of a bone and is often called a *hairline fracture* (see Fig. 3b). It is tough to diagnose, sometimes not showing up on X-rays during the first few weeks of the injury. By the time the fracture is detectable, the pain has already stopped and no more X-rays are taken, so it often continues to be undetected—perhaps causing trouble later.

(A most famous recent case was that of pro basketball

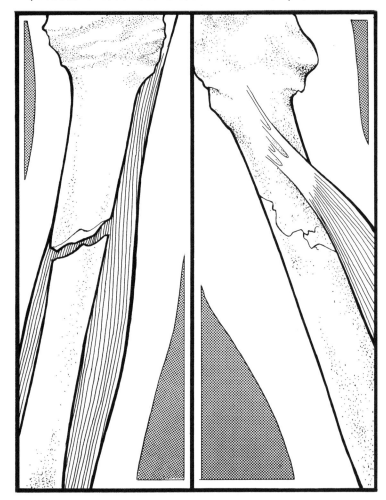

Fig. 3a. *A complete bone fracture can cause damage to the surrounding tissue if any stress is placed on it.*

Fig. 3b. *A stress fracture often goes completely undetected.*

star Bill Walton, who began suffering pain in his left foot in October of 1979, shortly after he had joined the San Diego Clippers. It was later diagnosed as a broken bone in the top of the foot, and he played only fourteen games that season. The season before he had played no games for the Portland Trail Blazers because of foot problems.

(It's difficult to imagine a sport that could be harder on an athlete's feet than pro basketball. National Basketball Association teams play more than eighty games a season, not counting exhibitions, playoffs, and almost daily practices. Up and down the courts the players run, up and down they leap for shots and rebounds. Thousands and thousands of times.)

Stress fractures usually don't require a cast, since the bone is already in its proper position. Training should stop until the break has healed, however, or it can lead to a complete break.

Stress fractures don't always come from a single, powerful impact. They can come from repeated stresses such as the pounding of the feet on pavement during long runs, or even from doing too many bench presses with too heavy a weight. Whatever the causes, you might have to change your training program to prevent similar injuries in the future. This might mean cushioning your heel more or progressing more slowly with your weight-training program.

YOUNGBLOOD AND THE LONE HORSEMAN

Caution, caution, and more caution has been advised in this section, but there are some tales of foolhardy heroism that are irresistible. Just don't try to imitate these particular heroes: Jack Youngblood, All-Pro defensive end for the Los Angeles Rams, and Ernie Nevers, a multi-sport star at Stanford University in the 1920s.

In a 1979 playoff game versus Dallas, Youngblood suffered a hairline fracture of his left fibula, about two inches above the ankle. Although it happened in the second quarter, he played in the rest of that game and in a subsequent playoff victory over Tampa Bay, plus Super Bowl XIV against Pittsburgh. For the last two games his leg was protected by a fiberglass cast.

"Why shouldn't I play?" he asked the press in a joking mood. "The bone isn't sticking out and there isn't any blood." And more seriously: "I trust our doctors implicitly. They told me there is no way to further injure the break, not with the precautions we're taking, the tape jobs, the supportive cast."

In fact, Youngblood did not further damage his leg, and he was back in action for the Rams in the 1980 season.

The 1925 Rose Bowl featured the famous Four Horsemen of Notre Dame, one of the greatest backfields ever: Don Miller, Elmer Layden, Jim Crowley, and Harry Stuhldreher. Stanford relied on Nevers, a blond bull from the Midwest. The trouble was, Nevers was recovering from two recently broken ankles.

With his legs tightly wrapped in bandages, tape, and part of an inner tube, Nevers played the whole game on defense and on offense carried the football 34 times for 114 yards. Luckily, he didn't permanently damage himself, for he went on to play both major-league baseball and football.

Oh, yes. Notre Dame won the game 27-10.

Damage to the Wrapper

The popular term "bone bruise" is technically inaccurate. The bone itself doesn't bruise; it's the cover or wrapping around the bone—the periosteum—that bruises from high impact.

Bone bruises are quite painful (in fact, it's usually the degree of pain that leads to the diagnosis), but they're quick to heal if left undisturbed. That means preventing additional blows similar to those which caused the injury in the first place. For example, if the bruise is on the bottom of the heel, it's best to stop running until the pain is gone. Continued running will only aggravate the injury.

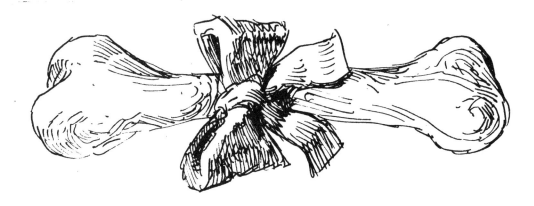

Tibia Tribulations

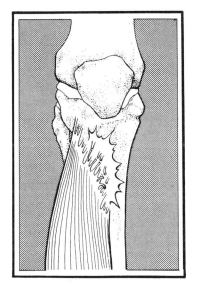

Fig. 4. *Shin Splints—tearing of the muscle-origin fibers from the tibia or fibula—are caused by running on hard surfaces.*

The tibia, more often called the shinbone, can become a painful trouble spot for basketball players and athletes who perform on hard surfaces (say, a city-streets jogger or a tennis player reared on California hardcourts). *Shin splints* is the name given to burning tibia pain during or after running and to tibia soreness the next day. According to *The Doctor's Guide to Better Tennis & Health*, shin splints are the "small tearing of muscle origin fibers from the tibia itself" (see Fig. 4) or from the membrane between the tibia and the other lower-leg bone, the fibula.

David Fechtman, trainer for the Association of Tennis Professionals, says that causes of the tearing include "falling arches, undue stress, muscle fatigue, constantly changing playing surfaces, and a lack of reciprocal muscle coordination" between the front and back parts of the lower leg.

If shin splints are hampering an athlete, Fechtman recommends four things he or she should do before a workout: take two aspirins, apply heat, stretch the muscles of the lower leg, and strap one-and-a-half-inch tape up to a width of three inches just above the ankle bone. After a workout, apply ice to the sore shinbone for up to ten minutes.

The Backbone Blues

The spine is an S-shaped column of thirty-three bones (vertebrae) that goes from the base of the skull down to the tailbone, or coccyx. The vertebrae form a tube or canal that protects the vital spinal cord and its membranes. Except for the lowest four, which are fused to form the coccyx, and the next five, also fused, each vertebra rests on the one below at an angle, held in place by muscles and ligaments, and is separated from its neighbors by shock absorbers called discs.

Damage to the spinal cord by injury or disease can cause paralysis of both legs (paraplegia). A severe neck injury can cause the victim to lose control of all limbs, becoming a quadriplegic. (Ex-UCLA volleyball All-America Kirk Kilgour broke his neck in a gymnastics accident in Europe. Today he coaches Pepperdine University's volleyball team from a wheelchair.) Unless he or she is in danger of drowning, a person suffering from a severe neck injury should be moved only by experts.

Most backbone injuries are not so ghastly. Frequently an athlete will crack a bony projection on a vertebra, which is quite painful. Such fractures can be diagnosed only by X-ray and are easily curable by rest and ice application. Back pain—which is frequent, for instance, among gymnasts who practice back-bends—should not be ignored, for fractures of the spine, if untreated, can lead to to *spondylolisthesis*, in which the whole spinal column slips forward.

Speaking of slippage, slipped discs and similar spinal ailments are usually caused by incorrect lifting. When lifting heavy objects, weightlifters and everybody else should bend their knees and let their legs do most of the work. Don't bend from the waist. (See Fig. 5.)

Other tips: alternate loads from one arm to the other; don't lift heavy objects over your head (it causes your spine to arch too much); don't sleep on your stomach (again, too much arch); and keep your weight down.

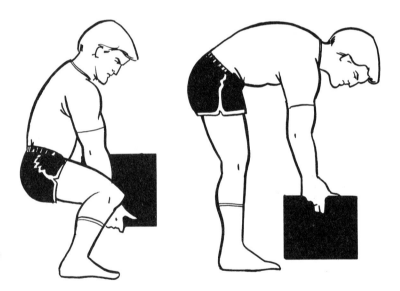

Fig. 5. *To prevent back injury, bend at the knees and let your legs carry the burden of lifting heavy objects.*

Tendon and Ligament Injuries

Torn Tendon Troubles

Picture the tendon as a more densely packed, stronger extension of the muscle, which it connects to a bone. Considering the small size of the tendon relative to the muscle (refer to Fig. 6), it's understandable why strong, healthy tendons are essential to good athletic performance. That comparatively diminutive tendon must carry all its muscle's force to the corresponding bone.

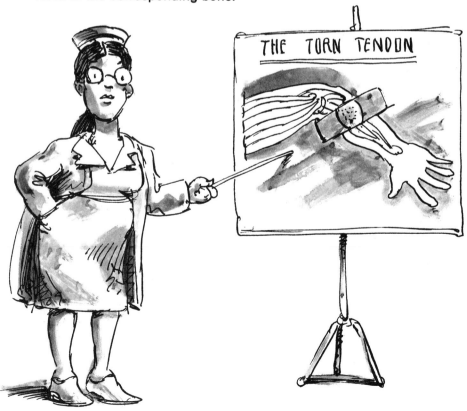

THE TORN TENDON

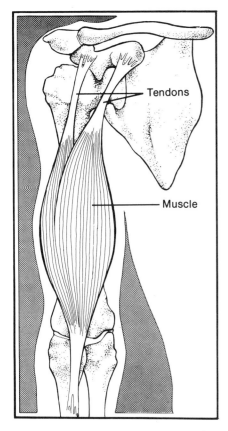

Fig. 6. *Tendon tears and ruptures can be prevented by warm-up exercises.*

Injury-prevention techniques are important in the protection of tendons. A flexibility and warm-up program takes only minutes of your training time while greatly reducing potential damage.

Tearing a tendon is like tearing a piece of fabric. A yard-wide fabric can be torn an inch or a yard. Likewise, a tendon can be torn a little or a lot. A tendon rupture is a tendon torn all the way into two pieces. Anything less than a rupture is termed a tear.

Tears and ruptures come from overloads—an extra stretch, a blow to an already stretched tendon, too much weight. Whatever the reason, the treatment is the same.

The article on emergency treatment (ice, compression, elevation, etc.) outlined the best method of treating tendon tears. The object is to reduce swelling, that difficult byproduct of most new injuries. If the tendon is ruptured—you can tell by your inability to contract the muscle—you must see a doctor. As is also true of a ruptured muscle, surgery is the *only way* to mend a completely torn tendon.

How to rehabilitate the damaged tendon depends on the extent of the injury. The same logic applies to treating a *torn* tendon as to treating a torn muscle, so follow the advice given in the section on treatment and rehabilitation.

Rehabilitating a *ruptured* tendon is more of an ordeal. After surgery, a cast is put on to prevent movement of the healing area. After the cast comes off, most physical trainers and therapists design a rehabilitation program that takes into consideration any muscle shrinkage created by lack of use. Weight training is often recommended. Specifics of the workouts are best left to a professional who understands the specific degree of the injury.

Tendinitis: Achilles Heel and Erving Knee

Julius Erving, the acrobatic all-star forward on the Philadelphia 76ers pro basketball team, ices his knees at *halftime* of games as well as afterward. Why? Tendinitis, an old enemy of athletes (sometimes spelled "tendonitis"). Achilles heel and jumper's knee are variations of this problem, which is inflammation of a tendon resulting from overuse, overstretching, or overloading. Basketball players, runners, dancers, and weightlifters are all likely victims because of the enormous stress they place on the tendons.

Tendinitis usually develops slowly. The athlete notices "a little soreness" during daily workouts. Unfortunately, continu-

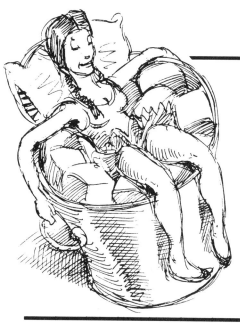

ing the workouts increases the pain and lengthens the eventual recovery time.

Complete rest is the most widely recommended treatment. But realistically, the competitive athlete's personality usually won't allow complete rest, so most try to keep the pain to a minimum rather than eradicate it altogether. Thus, Erving uses ice at halftime, which accomplishes that goal.

Some athletes have found that orthodiscs (individually prescribed shoe inserts) reduce or eliminate knee and ankle problems by redistributing the force on those areas. Professional treatment ranges from ultrasound to cortisone injections. (Caution: cortisone use should be one of the last resorts, because continued use can dissolve hard tissue within the treated area.)

Tennis Elbow: A Splendid Backhand (Ouch!) Down the Line

Tennis instructors insist that the backhand stroke is more natural than the forehand. Why? Because the forehand stroke actually begins *behind* your body and moves across it, whereas the backhand is executed from a more natural position perpendicular to your body and in front of it. Still, no matter what the experts claim, beginners continue to lack confidence in their backhands. And, worse, incorrectly hit backhands get most of the blame for that common, painful ailment, tennis elbow. ("Tennis elbow" is a general term covering quite a few possible maladies, but most of the time it refers to tendinitis.)

It's fine to have a short, punchy backhand stroke in Ping-Pong, and it's desirable to have a short, punchy backhand stroke when volleying at the net in tennis, but the regular tennis backhand for ground strokes should be fluid, with a thorough follow-through.

"Inferior players punch at the ball and fail to transfer their weight, putting great pressure on their arms," says Dr. Robert P. Nirschl of Georgetown University in Washington, D.C. ". . . I had tennis elbow until I began hitting a more fluid backhand. The backhand is what almost always causes tennis elbow."

There are two other causes, according to Stanford Coach . Dick Gould: gripping the racket too tightly and using excessive wrist roll or jerkiness in the forehand.

Elbow braces, cortisone shots, and even surgery have been used successfully to cure various kinds of tennis elbow, but rest is usually cure enough. And using proper, un-Ping-Pongy form on the backhand will prevent any more trouble.

Overstreeeeetched Ligaments

Marathon runner Bill Rogers steps in a hole while jogging across the Massachusetts countryside. Instead of all his weight coming down on a well-padded heel, for an instant it's on the side of his foot. His ankle twists, and he falls. Dallas Cowboys running back Tony Dorsett gets tackled from the right side just as he plants his right foot in the turf. When the pileup is untangled, he stays on the ground clutching his knee.

Both have suffered sprained, or overstretched, ligaments. As tendons hold muscles to bones, ligaments hold bones to bones at joints, much the same way as a door and frame are joined by a hinge.

Damage to the ligaments is more often than not a result of overstretching when the joint is twisted or pulled beyond its normal range of motion, as shown in Figure 7. Sporting events are packed with opportunities for overstretching, which can cause anything from a minor irritation to a catastrophe that demands surgery.

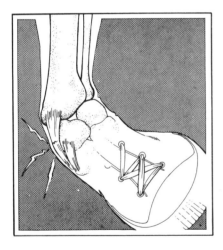

Fig. 7. *A sprained ligament occurs when a joint is twisted beyond its normal range.*

Whether mild or severe, "sprain" is the catch-all name for overstretched ligaments that aren't torn. For athletes, sprains are most common at the knees, ankles, or wrists. The symptoms: pain at a joint followed by swelling and discoloration. (There is some confusion caused by the general terms *sprain* and *strain*. Just remember that a sprain is a straining or wrenching of the parts around a joint, without dislocation. So all sprains are strains, but not all strains are sprains.)

Emergency treatment for a sprained ligament is exactly the same as for a strained muscle (see "The Iceman Cureth. . ."), the idea being to reduce swelling. And the same rehabilitation procedures should be followed after all pain has disappeared.

The ligament might be stretched so much that it tears—a few cells or all the way across (a rupture). A little bit of extra tear means lots of extra agony.

A mild tear is treated as and sometimes called a sprain. But a ruptured ligament requires professional care; surgery is the only way to join the pieces. Of course, treating the injury as an emergency during the first forty-eight hours will prevent unnecessary damage from swelling.

Joint Injuries

Dislocated Joints: Damage to the Body's Hinges

In November of 1980, basketball player Lonnie Shelton of the Seattle SuperSonics underwent a three-hour operation in a Seattle hospital to repair chronically dislocated bones in his left wrist. The cause was unknown, but the wrist was in such bad shape, said Dr. Edward Almquist, that there were no ligaments left!

Shelton is right-handed, so the problem didn't affect his shooting as much as it might have. Still, his left hand was his guiding hand in shooting and was needed to grip the ball on rebounds and catch passes. The surgical solution was to drill holes in the bones so that the dislocated ones could be lashed together. Shelton was declared out for the season, and Dr. Almquist said the

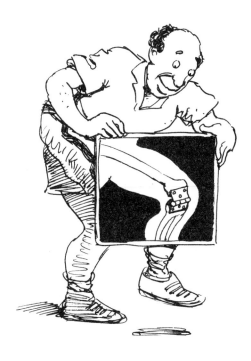

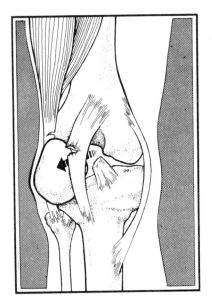

Fig. 8. *A dislocated joint can cause damage to the muscles, tendons, ligaments, and cartilage.*

four-year veteran from Oregon State might not ever regain full use of the wrist.

Shelton's was an unusual case. The more common areas for a dislocation (the end of a bone being displaced from a joint) are the shoulders, hips, elbows, fingers, and kneecaps. It usually happens when an athlete falls or receives a hard blow.

The most obvious outward indication is a deformed joint. Many basketball players have looked down to see one finger bone riding atop another after being jammed on the fingertip by an improperly caught ball.

Although the basketball player's first instinct might be to pull the dislocated digit straight with the other hand, the right thing to do is follow the guidelines in the first part of this section about emergency treatment. The jammed finger should be treated as a bone break rather than a dislocation. One can never be too cautious.

Rehabilitating a dislocated joint often requires more time and patience than rehabilitating other common athletic injuries. Why? The dislocation damages more things—muscles, tendons, ligaments, and cartilage (see Fig. 8). So a lot more has to heal.

"The Human Arm Is Not Built to Pitch a Baseball"

"Medial epicondyle" sounds like a prehistoric monster, but actually it's a part of the elbow that causes trouble for youngsters—the site of the dread affliction called "Little League elbow."

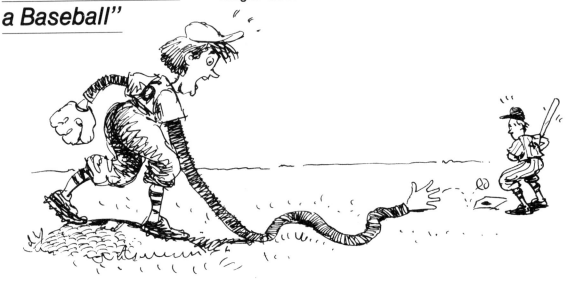

So, a quick anatomy lesson. The humerus is the upper arm bone. As you hold your arm straight out, with the palm of the hand up, the knob on the inner part of your elbow is the medial epicondyle of the humerus. In young boys and girls it is only weakly attached to the humerus.

Overwork and throwing curve balls are the two big culprits —the latter because of the twist of the wrist which puts strain on the elbow. Try giving your own throwing wrist a violent twist in either direction, and you'll get the idea. In the words of the famous orthopedic surgeon Dr. Robert Kerlan, "The human arm is not built to pitch a baseball."

The humerus and the epicondyle can separate because of constant pull of the attached forearm muscles from excessive throwing. And on the outside part of the elbow are the opposing ends of the humerus and one of the forearm bones. This is a less frequent trouble spot where bone chips might develop. Young pitchers can suffer osteochondritis, or erosion of the cartilage at the end of the bones comprising the elbow joint, resulting in loose chips in the joint and limitation of motion.

To avoid Little League elbow, here are some simple rules:

1. Don't ignore a young pitcher's elbow soreness.

2. Don't let him or her throw curves.

3. Don't let a young pitcher practice throwing at home, because, as an elbow expert has said, "Excessive throwing at this age invites trouble rather than perfection."

4. Don't let the season or the individual pitching stints go on too long.

5. Rear your kid to be a shortstop.

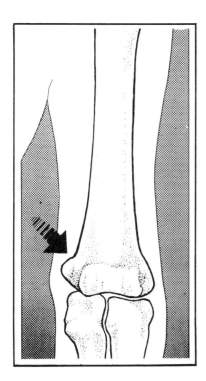

Fig. 9. *A few too many curveballs thrown by a young pitcher can cause Little League elbow.*

Water on the Knee

Synovia is not an Eastern European country next to Albania, but transparent membranes which encase the articulating parts of the joints (bones, tendons, cartilage) and reduce friction among them by secreting a lubricating fluid. Synovitis is an inflammation of a synovium, or synovial membrane. This inflammation can be caused by arthritis, various injuries, and various infections.

Synovitis in the knee, common among athletes, is accompanied by a painful swelling in which the kneecap floats on a

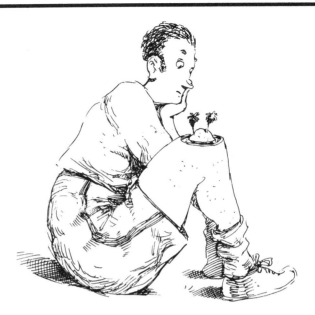

little lake of clear (synovial) fluid—thus the term "water on the knee." The pain restricts motion, which isn't so bad for a chess master but is terrible for a left tackle or a point guard.

Rest is the best cure, but sometimes the condition is so bad that the knee must be drained. Jack Curran, trainer of the Los Angeles Lakers basketball team, uses aspirin to ease the pain and drugs such as Butazolidin to reduce the inflammation, plus heat before the games and lots of ice afterward.

Bursitis: The Sad-Sac Malady

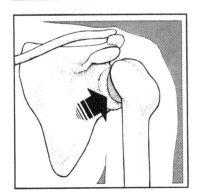

Fig. 10. *Inflammation of the bursa can cause painful friction whenever the affected joint moves.*

A bursa is not a Synovian handbag, but a fluid-filled sac, pouch, or cushion that helps ease the movement of a joint by preventing or minimizing friction. A shoulder bursa is shown in Figure 10. (Bursae is the plural form of the word.) Infection, injury, or unusual muscular effort can cause bursitis, the painful inflammation of a bursa.

Bursitis of the shoulder is obviously going to hamper a swimmer, quarterback, or racquetball player. Bursitis of the knee is going to hinder just about any athlete but a wheelchair basketball player. Rest is usually enough to cure it, but heat and massage can cut the pain in the meantime. Drugs must occasionally be used, and sometimes accumulated fluid and calcium salts must be drained.

(The Greeks, by the way, gave us the suffix *itis*, which is used to mean the inflammation of an organ. Hence come the words arthritis, neuritis, tendinitis, conjunctivitis, bursitis, *ad infinitum*.)

Shock-Absorber Problems

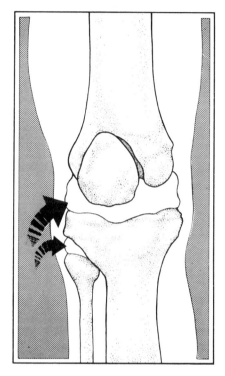

Fig. 11. *Cartilage provides a cushion between bones to absorb shock.*

Cartilage, or gristle, is the shock-absorbing connective tissue found between bones (see Fig. 11). It is a semi-transparent whitish or yellowish material that forms most of a shark's skeleton but very little of a human's. Cartilage pads between bones are often bruised or torn during the bang and crash of sports competition. The severity ranges from slightly discomforting to career-ending.

Symptoms vary from minor irritation to intense pain and swelling, depending on the seriousness of the injury. Many basketball players have knee pain because of the constant pounding the knee cartilage gets from repeated jumps. The force of the landing is equivalent to striking the cartilage with a hammer from the bottom.

Follow the previously outlined emergency treatment for any minor cartilage damage. The main objective is to keep the swelling away by using cold compresses, wrappings, and elevation of the injured joint. Swelling frequently damages more tissue than is hurt by the initial injury.

A suspected serious injury—a tear rather than a bruise, usually recognizable by extremely severe pain—requires a doctor's help. Surgery is often needed to mend the tear. You usually don't have to worry about an unnecessary operation because modern methods of diagnosis are quite accurate.

Rehabilitation varies depending on the type of injury. Basketball players often apply icebags to bruised, sore knee cartilage after every practice and are ready to resume training the following day. But torn cartilage, even with the best of medical care, usually means a minimum of twelve weeks off from serious workouts.

Skin Ailments

Fungi Are No Fun, or There's Mold in Them Thar Hills

Fungi—a division of plant life that includes mushrooms, toadstools, yeasts, and molds—flourish not only in soil but in many types of warm, damp places. That includes between human toes (athlete's foot) and in the human groin (jock itch). The fungi that cause these contagious diseases are parasites that are sometimes difficult to get rid of, especially during hot weather.

The disease-bearing fungi are particularly drawn to athletes because both host and unwanted guest happen to thrive, or at least function, in damp areas. Gang showers and sweaty uniforms—an athlete's regular, if only part-time, environment—provide ideal breeding grounds for fungi, which proliferate there and spread to the frequently damp bodies of the athletes themselves.

Athlete's foot starts with scaling and itching between the toes: then cracks or lesions appear and become sore. The condition can spread to the tops or bottoms of the feet and cause serious

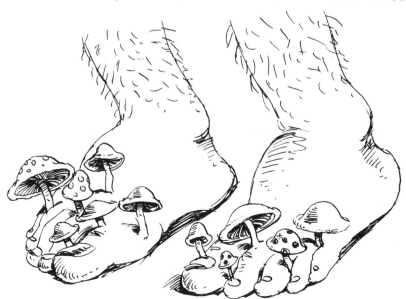

problems if not attended to promptly. Drugstores have many nonprescription creams and powders that are usually effective against athlete's foot.

Two good ways to prevent having your feet become fungus farms: Dry carefully between your toes after showering, and change socks every day.

There are also plenty of non-prescription cures for jock itch (which can occur under women's breasts, too). Prevention tips: keep the area as clean and dry as possible and change underwear frequently.

(All of the above maladies are forms of ringworm, which has nothing at all to do with worms but is merely a ghastly catch-all name for contagious skin diseases caused by parasitic fungi.)

The Gunk

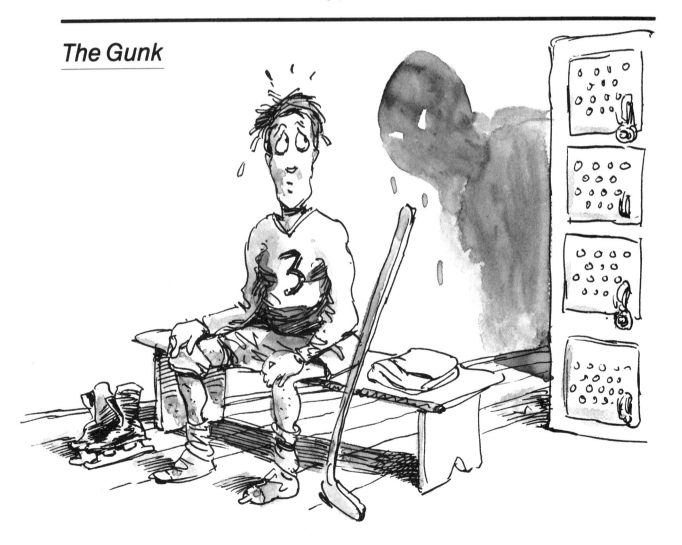

One of the nastiest occupational hazards in sports is a rash nicknamed "the gunk," which has tormented many ice hockey players since the early 1970s. Most who suffer from it are merely uncomfortable (about 10 percent of the National Hockey League players are affected at any one time), but a few have been hospitalized because of it, and one, defenseman Tom Reid of the NHL's Minnesota North Stars, was forced to retire.

"In 1975 I noticed it on my hands," he said. "Then my skin cracked wide open all over my body, and a yellowish fluid oozed out. I had to quit playing hockey because I couldn't sleep anymore. The liquid would ooze out and stick to the sheets when I slept. When I moved, it would tear my skin off. Finally I had to sleep without any clothes, sitting up in a wooden chair. I just couldn't go on living like that."

Reid sued Lloyd's of London, the NHL's disability insurer, for $165,000 in accident disability payments.

What causes the gunk? Dermatologists disagree. One promising theory is that microscopic fiberglass particles from hockey sticks become embedded in players' underwear and rub against the skin. Other theories: synthetic materials used in padding and underwear cause allergic reactions; the gunk is just an exaggerated heat rash; stress is to blame; filthy conditions in NHL visitors' locker rooms are wonderful breeding grounds for all types of germs. (Since fiberglass sticks became popular in the league about the same time the disease appeared, and since hockey players do indeed love to sand and hone their sticks, the fiberglass-particle theory has some strong support.)

Dr. William Schorr of Marshfield, Wisconsin, has advanced the idea that the gunk really is several different skin ailments: "I think the combination of friction from wearing pads, sweating heavily, and playing in arenas with high humidity causes many of these problems."

Whatever the cause, the gunk has not reared its rashy head in pro football—our other sport featuring well-padded gladiators. The National Football League had a brief problem with artificial turf dye causing skin rashes, but that was easily solved by changing the chemical composition of the dye.

Drugs for Injuries

Aspirin and Beyond

Pain is an unavoidable consequence of sports. St. Louis Cardinals first baseman Keith Hernandez stretches too far to take a throw and "pulls" a groin muscle. Chicago Bears quarterback Vince Evans gets hit a certain way by a tackler or two and suffers a hyperextended knee. Golfer Donna Caponi spends too much time on the practice tee and develops a sore shoulder. A common way to eliminate, reduce, or mask pain is by taking a drug.

Aspirin is far and away the most common pain-relieving, or analgesic, drug—and not just for athletes. An estimated one hundred million aspirin tablets are swallowed in America every day! (Many products using aspirin are known by brand names—Anacin, Bufferin, Alka-Seltzer. But in the U.S. the word aspirin is generic, or not protected by trademark registration.) Its popularity is warranted, for a study at the famous Mayo Clinic in Minnesota concluded that ". . . Among all analgesics and narcotics available for oral use, none have been demonstrated to show a consistent advantage over aspirin for the relief of any type of pain."

How does aspirin make an ache go away? It cuts down the concentration in the tissues of chemicals (prostaglandins) that help produce inflammation and pain. It also reduces fever by causing the dilation of blood vessels in the skin, which in turn hurries the loss of body heat. And it reduces blood clotting, which means it's bad for people with ulcers or excessive bleeding (hemophilia).

Some other common pain-relievers:

Darvon, Darvon Compound, Harmar (propoxyphene): A prescription drug probably not as effective as aspirin in many cases. One book, *The People's Pharmacy*, by Joe Graedon (St. Martin's Press), calls it an "overrated pain-killer that has been highly promoted."

Codeine: Introduced in 1886, thirteen years before aspirin, this prescription drug relieves moderate pain but can also cause drowsiness, constipation, and lightheadedness. Many cough remedies contain it.

Percodan, Percobarb (oxycodone): A mild prescription analgesic taken in tablet form. It works much like codeine and is used to relieve pain and coughing. "Percs" are said to be popular in some pro football circles.

Talwin (pentazocine): A mild prescription painkilling tablet. Some athletes are popping Talwin before performing in hopes that their pain thresholds will be raised. Although scientists are uncertain about how it works, some athletes believe it prevents news of pain from getting to the brain from the exhausted or damaged body. Although not in a league with injecting heroin, of course, taking Talwin *before* an event is drug abuse.

Demerol (meperidine): A strong prescription analgesic introduced more than forty years ago. Scientists are not absolutely certain how it works.

Butazolidin (phenylbutazone): A mild prescription drug that acts against pain, fever, and inflammation. "Bute" is often used to treat hurting racehorses. Jockeys are not thrilled by that; they believe an ailing horse doctored with Bute might break down in the midst of a race, fall, and perhaps get a few animals and humans badly hurt or killed.

Warning: Some of these drugs are habit-forming, some cause serious problems when the athlete is taking other drugs, some cause mild-to-horrendous allergic reactions. See a doctor before swallowing, inserting, or injecting.

The Solvent that Stifles Pain

DMSO (dimethyl sulfoxide) is a bad-tasting, foul-smelling industrial solvent, a byproduct of wood chips during the manufacture of plain brown paper. It is also a popular, effective, liniment-like pain-killer, which—according to a New York osteopath—is "so widespread, there's not a professional sports team or dance company that doesn't use it."

"DMSO has the largest potential number of uses ever documented for a single chemical," says Dr. Stanley Jacob, a surgeon at the University of Oregon Health Sciences Center in Portland. "There's nothing like it."

"Everybody uses DMSO," says distance runner Alberto Salazar, winner of the 1980 New York Marathon.

"When guys get hurt they come to me [for DMSO] before they go to the trainer," said backup quarterback June Jones of the Atlanta Falcons, an enthusiastic DMSO proponent. "It's tremendous on [turf] burns."

The trouble is, DMSO is illegal for medical use (except for a certain type of bladder disorder) in all but three states: Florida, Louisiana, and Oregon. The Food and Drug Administration outlawed it in 1965 because it had caused eye damage in lab animals, yet veterinarians have used it legally for years. Recently the FDA warned that the chemical can cause skin rashes and, if contaminated, carry poisons through the skin and into the body.

There is lots of controversy over the drug, an eight-ounce bottle of which is sold on the black market for $20 and up. Some pro-DMSO people have charged that major drug com-

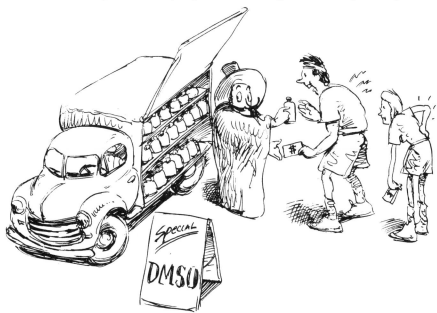

panies don't want to see the chemical approved by the FDA because Crown Zellerbach, the big paper manufacturer, owns the patent for its use as a pain-killer. A legal DMSO, say its boosters, would severely cut into sales of pain-killers already on the market.

Here's an example of what's been going on:

A school superintendent in the state of Washington ordered the Crescent High School football team in Port Angeles to stop using DMSO to heal bruises. Athletes at that school had been swabbing the solvent on bruises for ten years, according to football coach Gary Kautz. "Most top college and pro teams use it and maybe three-quarters of the high school teams in the state," says Kautz.

"The first time I used it, my legs went numb for five minutes," says an 18-year-old football player. "But it helps with pain and playing with bruises."

Cortisone Can Be Worse than the Disease

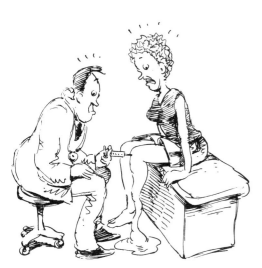

Cortisone is a steroid hormone produced by the outer walls of the adrenal glands, located just above the kidneys. All healthy people have some of it circulating in their bodies. Levels are higher when they're working hard or under stress, as natural cortisone is the body's healing agent. In many ways, it's a first cousin to adrenaline.

Scientists have learned how to make synthetic cortisone, or they can take it from the adrenal glands of certain domesticated animals. It reduces or eliminates inflammation, so it is often injected into the joints to battle such ailments as rheumatoid arthritis, bursitis, and tendinitis.

Synthetic cortisone has become a commonly overused pain reliever for athletes' joint problems—tennis elbow, for one. But few know that continued injections in a joint can soften the hard materials there. For example, too many cortisone injections in the knee can actually dissolve the kneecap and end a promising career.

Overdosage or prolonged use of cortisone may cause water retention (which in turn may cause facial swelling, or "moon face"), high blood pressure, facial hair on females, and even mental disorder.

Children should definitely *not* have cortisone shots in the weight-bearing joints—ankles, knees, hips. Rest usually cures the ailing joints of kids anyway.

Substances that Injure the Athlete

Alcoholism: "An Equal-Opportunity Disease"

Norm Standlee was a six-foot-two-inch, 230-pound fullback on the great Stanford "Wow Boys" football team of 1940 —the team credited with popularizing the T-formation. Later he fought in World War II and played professional football for the Chicago Bears and San Francisco 49ers. Handsome and popular, he seemed destined to enjoy a happy, successful life.

Instead, Standlee made himself, his family, and his many friends unhappy because of his addiction to booze. He died alone at age sixty-two in Room 212 of the EZ-8 Motel, not far from the Stanford campus. Cause of death: cirrhosis of the liver, brought on by alcoholism. For the last four years of his sad life he had been in and out of hospitals, sanitariums, and motels. Near the end, Standlee would be waiting every morning at eleven when the bartender arrived to open the restaurant/bar next to the EZ-8.

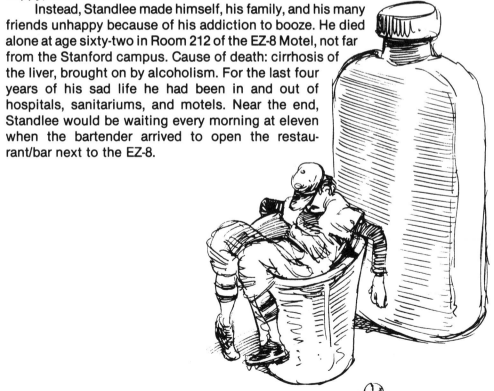

Liquor is a drug that not only hinders athletic performance, as discussed earlier in "Save the Alcohol for the Rubdown Table," but ruins lives as well. Athletes, of course, are not immune. Wrestler Gorgeous George, pitcher Ryne Duren, ex-USF basketball All-America Don Lofgran (who died in a Salt Lake City hotel room in much the same circumstances as Standlee)—all had serious drinking problems.

"Alcoholism is an equal-opportunity disease," says Dr. Keith Simpson, president of the National Council on Alcoholism. "One out of every ten people catches alcoholism. It is chronic and progressive."

The Los Angeles Dodgers, perhaps the best-run franchise in sports, has started an alcohol rehabilitation program, run by ex-pitcher Don Newcombe, the club's director of community relations. Newk was another who drank too much for too long.

"My baseball career came to an end when I was 32 years old," he said. "Had these programs been available at that time and had somebody been paying attention to it, the baseball career of Don Newcombe could have been extended another four or five years."

With the help of Newcombe and the Dodgers, pitcher Bob Welch, twenty-three, checked into an alcoholic treatment center in Arizona and stayed five weeks. At the following spring training, he told his teammates and the press that he was an alcoholic and was battling the problem. Not long after, Kansas City Royals catcher Darrell Porter admitted that he had been not only an alcoholic but also a frequent user of other drugs. He, too, sought and received help from a rehabilitation center.

Just when does someone slip over the line from heavy drinker to alcoholic? According to Dr. Mark Keller of the Rutgers University Center of Alcohol Studies, it's when he or she "cannot consistently choose whether or not to drink" and, once boozing, "cannot consistently choose when to stop."

Smoking: Light Up for a Down Performance

"Cigarette smoking is the greatest preventable cause of illness, disability, and premature death in this country."

The surgeon general of the United States made that statement more than a decade ago, and it holds true today. Virtually every reputable scientist and physician in the nation says that tobacco users, in addition to having stained fingers, stained teeth, and bad breath, are much more likely than non-smokers to suffer from heart disease, respiratory ailments, and various types of cancer.

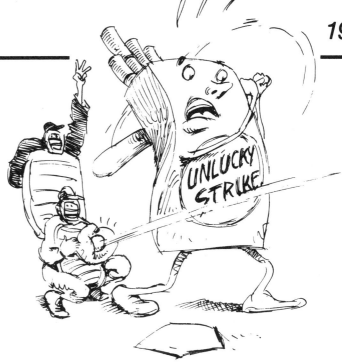

Smoking is also a hindrance to good athletic performance, especially in events and sports that require cardiovascular endurance. There are many reasons, but one of the main ones is that cigarette smoke contains carbon monoxide, which reduces the oxygen-carrying capacity of the blood (see the essay "Bogged Down by Smog," in the early part of this book). In *The Complete Book of Running*, James Fixx says, "As little as fifteen puffs of a cigarette can cause a 31-percent decrease in the body's oxygen-handling ability."

Also, smoking interferes with the process that removes particles of dust, soot, etc., from the bronchial tubes of the lungs. And it promotes the clogging and eventual *plugging* of the vessels that feed blood to the heart.

(Honus Wagner, a star baseball player for the Pittsburgh Pirates in the early part of this century, was opposed to cigarettes. So when the American Tobacco Trust came out with a Honus Wagner baseball card to be distributed as a premium with its cigarettes, the shortstop kicked up a fuss. The card was quickly taken out of circulation, but a few got out. One of those cards in good condition is worth more than $5,000 today, when most baseball cards come in bubble-gum packages.)

More than a few of today's pro baseball players are known to retreat from the dugout to the tunnel leading to the locker room for a quick smoke between innings. In endurance sports, however, serious competitors tend to stay away from cigarettes—at least those of the tobacco variety.

The Uppers Story

Amphetamines are stimulant drugs, or "uppers," which affect the user in much the same way as caffeine. Like caffeine—only much more so—the amphetamines provide a temporary feeling of well-being, reduce hunger, mask fatigue, and create the illusion of limitless energy and power. So they have a certain appeal to pleasure seekers, dieters, students staying up late to "cram" for exams . . . and athletes. Uppers, also called "speed" or "meth," are marketed under such brand names as Benzedrine, Dexedrine, and Methylamphetamine.

Inside the body, the action of amphetamines is similar to that of cocaine, which comes from the South American coca plant. Both drugs cause the release of a hormone from the brain (norepinephrine) and block its return to the storage sites. The brain centers sensitive to this hormone then cause the release of other hormones in the body.

There are no physical withdrawal symptoms when a person stops taking amphetamines, but he or she *can* become a psychically hooked pillhead. After only a short time—three to six days—of constant use, a stronger dose is needed to produce the desired effects. And then stronger.

An athlete who overdoses on uppers can suffer prolonged sleep loss, mental disturbance (persecution complex, forgetfulness, delusions of grandeur), and even death via heat prostration or high blood pressure. There is a period of depression or "crash" when the drug is stopped.

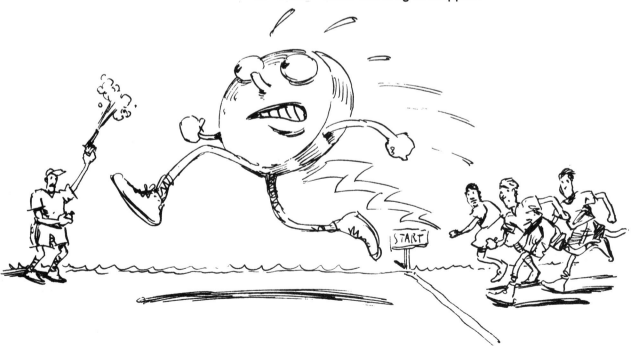

Hal Connolly, former Olympic Gold Medal winner in the hammer throw, says use of amphetamines is widespread among track-and-field athletes, except when (as at the Olympic Games) they know that post-competition testing will be administered.

"Cocaine is also becoming a popular performance stimulant," Connolly continues. "Athletes say if they take less than forty milligrams, it can't be traced and it gives a good boost for about three minutes."

Major-league catcher Darrell Porter, discussed in the article on alcohol, also had a cocaine habit, which cost him more than $1,000 a week, and took speed. He said the drugs made him paranoid: "Nine months ago I couldn't go shopping in a supermarket because I was so paranoid. When I was out driving, I was sure there was an army after me."

Downers

Athletes who depend regularly on uppers to spark their athletic performances usually find that the resulting "manic" feelings and behavior have an unwelcome overlap into their personal lives off the field or court. In order to rest, sleep, or just calm down, they often resort to the use of barbiturates.

Aptly called "downers," these intoxicant drugs come in more than twenty-five hundred forms and are marketed under such names as Luminal, Seconal, and Nembutal—all of which

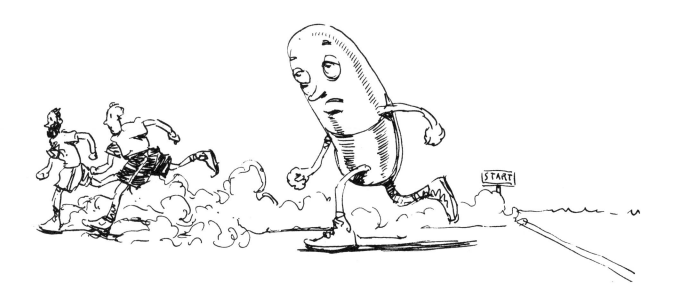

depress (slow down) the sleep-center nerves much as alcohol does. And they are as habit-forming as alcohol. After a while, the user has to swallow more and more to get to sleep; upon waking up, he or she experiences a period of mental depression and—especially bad for an athlete—slowed muscular performance. It soon becomes "necessary" for the pillhead to gear back up again with amphetamines—and the rollercoaster ride is on.

Combinations of alcohol, amphetamines, and barbiturates are extremely dangerous. Mr. or Ms. Habitprone gets high on speed, comes down and gets sleepy on booze and/or downers, forgets that he or she has taken a load of mind-numbers, and swallows more. Frequently the mixing of pills and alcohol keeps Habitprone down forever.

New Horizons

A Different Kind
of Needling

Acupuncture is a word derived from Latin (*acus* means needle, *punctura* means pricking), but it is also the name for an ancient Chinese medical practice, the origins of which are lost in oriental antiquity. The idea is to cure illness and reduce or eliminate pain by inserting sharp needles into specified parts of the body.

Today these needles, which can be up to four inches long, are made of stainless steel, with copper or aluminum handles. The needles can be inserted to various depths and at various angles. They can be rotated, left sticking in the skin for a while, or taken out immediately. It all depends on the ailment and the acupuncture expert's experience.

In America, acupuncture is not yet widely used in sports medicine, but it's no rarity. For instance, basketball player Kareem Abdul-Jabbar

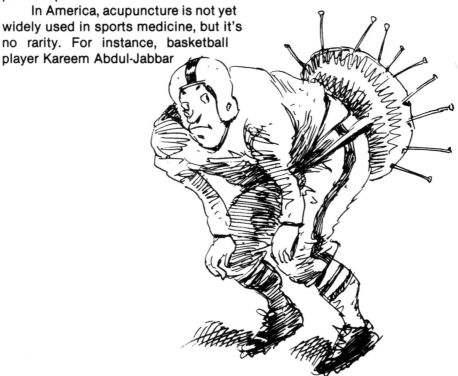

subjected himself to needling to reduce or remove the pain from the migraine headaches which have plagued him for years. It helped, but he recently returned to more traditional medicine to treat the headaches.

Other prominent athletes who have used acupuncture with some degree of success: quarterback Roman Gabriel (sore arm), linebacker Ed Lothamer (sore lower back), pitchers Dave LaRoche and Sam McDowell (sore arms), University of Kentucky running back Sonny Collins (sore knee). The needling has also been used on horses. One animal needler was described in a 1977 issue of *Sports Illustrated*: Dr. Paul Schmaltz of the Albuquerque Animal Acupuncture Clinic.

"When you talk to people about acupuncture, they don't believe it, and I don't blame them," said Dr. Schmaltz. "But acupuncture is perfect for racehorses. I give a horse a general treatment the day before a race. By post time the horse is feeling supergood. Its ears are up, its eyes are open, and you can hardly keep it on the ground." (Mobil Oil's famous flying red horse must have its own acupuncturist.)

Why does acupuncture work, at least in some cases? One theory is that each area of the skin's surface has a corresponding area in the brain. That also would account for the beneficial effects of massage.

Going in the Tank

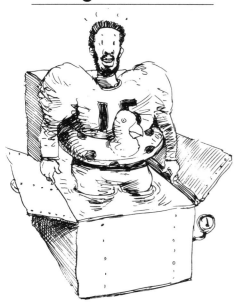

The Philadelphia Eagles pro football team was a big success in the 1980–81 playoffs, reaching the Super Bowl before losing to the Oakland Raiders. Perhaps some of the good performances were due to players "going in the tank," an expression which used to mean purposely losing a fight or game but which now has a completely different meaning in Philly.

The Eagles bought a $2,900 Float-to-Relax tank, an isolation chamber partially filled with a heated (93-94°F.) tap-water-and-salt solution. The tank is four feet wide, eight feet long, and four feet deep—impossibly claustrophobic for some. A player can loll in the enclosed, darkened tank and listen to classical or popular music tapes, self-hypnosis tapes (on relaxation, forgetting aches and pains, etc.), or nothing at all.

"I'm an intense person, and the tank really relaxes me," said linebacker Bill Bergey. "I don't think of anything in particular when I'm in it. My mind goes blank. It's great to float Sunday morning before a game."

"The tank is no panacea, and it won't cure you," trainer Otho Davis told the *Philadelphia Daily News*. "But if we can help an individual to relax and get his mind off his problems, then it's worth quite a bit."

An amateur athlete who can't afford the Float-to-Relax tank might get similar results by installing a hot-tub in his backyard and playing records or tapes from his own collection while he soaks.

From Russia with Energy

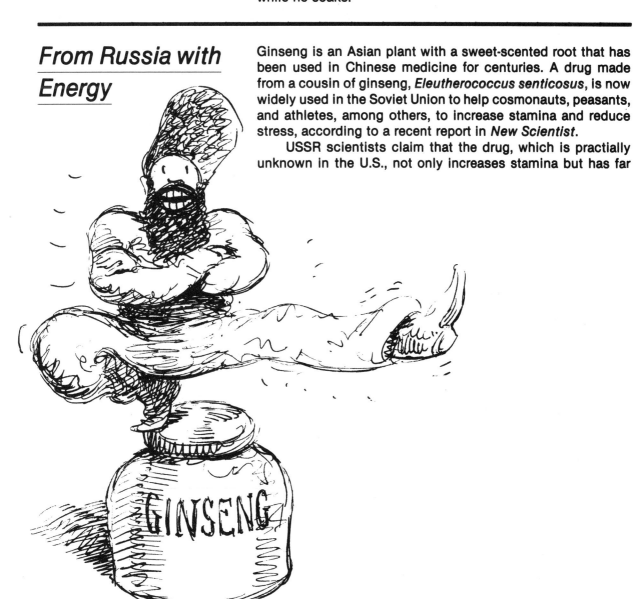

Ginseng is an Asian plant with a sweet-scented root that has been used in Chinese medicine for centuries. A drug made from a cousin of ginseng, *Eleutherococcus senticosus*, is now widely used in the Soviet Union to help cosmonauts, peasants, and athletes, among others, to increase stamina and reduce stress, according to a recent report in *New Scientist*.

USSR scientists claim that the drug, which is practially unknown in the U.S., not only increases stamina but has far fewer side effects than caffeine or any other known stimulant. "The only side effect was an occasional and transient rise in blood pressure," said the article's author, Dr. Stephen Fulder. And eleutherococcus apparently improves concentration.

Fulder cites a test conducted at the Lesgraft Institute of Physical Culture in Moscow. Eleutherococcus was given to a large group of athletes before a ten-mile run. Other athletes received placebos (substances that, unknown to them, would have no effect). The athletes who took the extract averaged about five minutes faster than the athletes who didn't.

BUT—there's always a catch, right?—it's sensible to be wary of wonder drugs. Until "eleuth" is carefully tested by the U.S. Food and Drug Administration (no one is quite sure *how* or *why* it works), ambitious athletes should not smuggle any home after vacationing in Siberia.

Index